6 *Myths*
About
Alternative Medicine

6 *Myths*
About
Alternative Medicine

*Using
It
Wisely*

Colleen C. Badell, Ph.D.

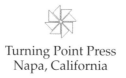

Turning Point Press
Napa, California

Turning Point Press
P.O. Box 4111
Napa, California 94558–0411

Copyright © 2006 by Colleen C. Badell, Ph.D.

All rights reserved.
Published 2006 by Turning Point Press.

No part of this book may be reproduced or transmitted in any form or by any means, electronic or mechanical, including photocopying, recording, or by any information storage and retrieval system, without permission in writing from the publisher.

Printed in the United States of America

For more information, visit www.health-advocate.com

Interior typesetting by Desktop Miracles
Index by Linzer Indexing Services
Cartoons rendered by Erin Leong

Library of Congress Control Number 2004098453
ISBN 0–9761129–1–4

CIP data available

The author has made every effort to ensure the accuracy of information contained in the book and to give credit reference material. Any omissions or errors are entirely unintentional.

Examples contained in this book are versions of actual consumer occurrences derived from clinical case files and first-hand accounts of events and circumstances. Names, locations, and other identifying data have been intentionally omitted to preserve the anonymity and protect the privacy of those involved.

CONTENTS

Preface   7

Introduction The History Behind the Myths   13

MYTH 1 The Healer Always Knows Best   25

MYTH 2 It Can't Hurt You   47

MYTH 3 All Remedies Are Created Equal   71

MYTH 4 You Can't Use It Without Proof   91

MYTH 5 It's a Good Substitute for
Conventional Medicine   113

MYTH 6 Spirit is Always Positive   143

Conclusion   165

Bibliography   171

Index   171

PREFACE

When I first began using alternative medicine in the early 1970s, it was not very popular. In fact, people who used it were frequently the object of ridicule and derision. In the past, those of us who braved the untried alternative medicine waters did so because, above all else, we believed in its effectiveness. Not only was the use of alternative medicine socially unacceptable for the consumer, but it was also economically unprofitable for the health care provider.

This environment has drastically changed. Today, alternative medicine is now both popular *and* profitable. The genesis for this book arose from this hotly competitive and lucrative marketplace.

The dramatic growth of alternative medicine practices and providers has made it more available to people than ever before. The potential for harm from using it has also increased exponentially. There are alternative practices with little or no value and alternative providers who are unskilled or who will misrepresent what their practices can do for you.

Although they existed in the early days of alternative medicine, disreputable practices and providers were much easier to discern than they are today. Packaging is more streamlined, and promotion is slicker than it ever was before. In this market, it has become increasingly difficult to tell fact from fiction, the real from the unreal.

As a longtime advocate and consumer of alternative medicine, I am concerned that we are not being educated about how to use it in the manner it was originally intended to be used and to its maximum potential. We use alternative medicine generically without consideration for all aspects of health and as a quick fix for our symptoms, much like we use conventional medicine. Alternative medicine, however, is totally different from conventional medicine— that's why it's called "alternative." We need to use it with a different attitude and approach than we use for conventional medicine.

Due to our natural inclination to use alternative medicine with a conventional approach, several

Preface

myths about it linger in the marketplace, which are perpetuated by many sources including health professionals, manufacturers of alternative products, and of course, the media. Some of these misconceptions result from our own mistaken beliefs, but others are encouraged by those who stand to gain financially from our belief in them. Public discourse on these issues is carefully avoided by leaders in the alternative medicine community, but what remains undiscussed can never be remedied.

Perhaps health professionals don't raise these issues because they fear that any criticism of alternative medicine, however constructive, will discourage its use at a time when its widespread acceptance is so tenuous, giving opponents fuel for the fire, so to speak. I take the opposite viewpoint. Dispelling these myths will only serve to encourage the wise use of alternative medicine and improve its chance of success, thereby increasing its acceptance into mainstream medicine.

There are six basic myths that influence our use of alternative medicine. Many of us still believe that the doctor knows best, so it's easy for us to apply this belief to alternative healers. We approach alternative medicine as the stereotypical passive and compliant health care consumer rather than adopt the involved and activist approach that alternative medicine requires.

Alternative medicine is often described as "natural" and "gentle," so our expectation is that any medicine this benevolent can't possibly hurt us, even though it may not do us any good. There are also hundreds of variations of the same alternative remedy or herb on the market. We assume that the herb St. John's Wort is the same regardless of the manufacturer or the manufacturing process.

A prevalent but controversial belief about alternative medicine, held by both alternative and conventional providers, is that you can't use it unless it has been proven effective by scientific study. Because science holds such prominence in our lives and our decision-making process, few of us are willing to consider the possibility that what it can do for us in the first place is extremely limited. (See John Horgan's *The End of Science.*)

Most of us take for granted that there is no adverse effect from applying an Eastern medical practice to a Western culture that approaches health and healing in very different ways. But when you try to fit one medicine into another medicine's paradigm, you are merely substituting one medicine for the other.

Spirit has become the new catch word for everything that is positive and wonderful about our lives. We have used and overused this word in all its forms and variations to the point at which its true meaning is diminished or lost altogether. In a commercialized world, everything is commodified and spirit is no exception to this rule. In the mistaken belief that it can be acquired, accumulated,

Preface

bought, or sold, spirit has been transformed into an object of desire and envy, over which we ardently compete. To some, it has become more a hobby than a state of mind, not unlike collecting stamps. Spirit is certainly not the former, but feeling good about yourself, being positive about life, and having a loving attitude are only part of the picture.

All of these myths about alternative medicine are intertwined and interconnected, affecting each other in numerous ways. Some of them are easy to understand, and some are more controversial. But they are all important, each in their own way.

Within each myth, there are also other common misconceptions, such as providers and medicines heal people, you have little control over your health, all alternative medicine is bad, alternative remedies are completely unregulated, and good medicine produces immediate results.

I want to address these myths, so the benefits of using alternative medicine can be maximized. In order to do this, the complexities of health care must be simplified into terms that are easily understood. In doing this, we can dispel the myth that understanding the nature of our health and the medicine that facilitates it is simply beyond us.

A better understanding of any medicine necessitates putting it into a broader context and forces us to examine the manner in which we approach our health. Once this is accomplished, specific steps can be taken to navigate the alternative medicine waters more safely, responsibly, and effectively. Practical suggestions are offered throughout the guide to assist in this endeavor.

Maintaining a state of health in an increasingly hazardous environment is a formidable task. Our environment is replete with toxic elements—physical, mental, and spiritual. The greatest challenge for us today is to deal with these elements within the limitations of a technology-based commercialized and institutionalized health care system. The availability of alternative medicine options makes this prospect a little easier. Alternative medicine is a medicine of great value and promise if we learn to use it wisely.

This book is intended not only for people who want to make better use of alternative medicine but also for those who want to empower themselves and assume a more active role in their own care. It is for people who are seeking greater meaning in illness and wellness and who are willing to regard all health challenges as supreme opportunities for learning and growth.

INTRODUCTION

The History
Behind the Myths

*An organism that destroys its
environment destroys itself.*

GREGORY BATESON

The trichotomy between the physical, mental, and
spiritual has only emerged in recent centuries and
coincides with the domination of a patriarchal point
of view and the subjugation of the sacred feminine.
Previous to this period in history, separation of the
physical, mental, and spiritual did not exist, and
everything was believed to be sacred by indigenous
cultures and ancient religious traditions.

This separation process began long ago. The Dark
Ages of ancient Egyptian and Greek medical practice
gave way to the Age of Reason in Greek and Roman

civilizations, which led to the European Renaissance of the fifteenth and sixteenth centuries. This marked a transitional period in which a traditionally spiritual perspective toward health was applied to an emerging secular science.

Out of this environment arose the development of science-based medicine. In its infancy, Western medicine continued to be concerned with healing both the body and soul and included the celestial sciences, such as astrology and metaphysics, in its practice. In the sixteenth and seventeenth centuries, the Italian astronomer and physicist Galileo, French mathematician and philosopher Descartes, and English mathematician and philosopher Sir Isaac Newton were all credited in varying degrees with the development of science in the West.

Science-based medicine focused solely on the physical because the all-powerful Catholic Church would only allow the practice of science as long as it was restricted to the physical. The mental and spiritual realms remained the province of the Church.

As science continued to evolve in the seventeenth century, man began to regard himself as separate from the living systems that surrounded him. The decline of feudalism in Western culture and rise of Protestantism resulting from Martin Luther's split with the Catholic Church encouraged the belief that man could master his own destiny. Earth became secular and equated with life, and

Introduction: The History Behind the Myths

heaven became sacred and equated with death. Earth and heaven were separate realms, and man was separate from them both. Man feared death as a separate entity associated with heaven and attempted to dominate and control earth in order to defy it, believing that he could remain unaffected by his actions.

A new paradigm arose from this perspective, which prized conquest and opposition and focused on the external causes of phenomena. This paradigm was the basis for modern scientific thought and investigation.

Out of man's belief in the separateness and singularity of life arose an irreverence for all living things. This irreverence bred the idea of disposability—since there is only one life to live, make the most of it regardless of the cost to ourselves or others. Everything is expendable when it comes to our own self-interest. This irreverence also encouraged the notion of duplicability—since there is no inherent nature to things, they can be recreated at will and without consequence. It is this detached point of view that caused the abandonment of the holistic healing methods of the past and gave rise to the secularized medicine of today.

In the nineteenth century, three other major events influenced the development of modern medicine. Charles Darwin's theory of evolution argued that all species, including human beings, had evolved over time. This controversial theory was a direct challenge to the religious view that God created man and continued to encourage the separation of the physical from the mental and spiritual. The Industrial Revolution was also born out of a scientific view of the physical world and was witness to the advent of technology and subsequent rise of mass culture. Promoting the idea that bigger, more, and faster were better, technology was utilized in medicine to eradicate the acute, killer diseases of the century.

Lastly, as a result of the exclusion of the mind from medical practice, a new science was created by a group of European medical doctors, which was termed psychology, or the science of the mind. Psychology concerned itself with the study of the mind separate from the body instead of integrating itself into the whole of medicine. Diseases of the mind were diagnosed as separate entities from diseases of the body with no connection to one another. Medicine and psychology were competing sciences rather than cooperative partners in the common goal of biological health.

With the fall of the omnipotent Catholic Church and its dominating spiritual influence, capitalism became the secular religion of the Western world. Capitalism promoted the institutionalization and commercialization of a technology-based medicine. The secularization of medicine reduced the role of the mental to the placebo treatment effect and relegated the spiritual to prima facie evidence

Introduction: The History Behind the Myths

of mental weakness or illness. Both the mind and spirit were regarded with suspicion and were dismissed by medical science as having little or no bearing on our physical health.

The advent of bodymind medicine acknowledged the impact of the mental on our physical health, but the care of our souls, once an inseparable part of every ancient healing tradition, continues to be more or less confined to the Sunday morning church service.

The Absence of Intimacy

In seeking to conquer our destiny by attempting to control the forces around us, we have inadvertently created a technologically advanced but spiritually bereft society. Where there is spiritual bereftment, there is an absence of intimacy, which some term "loss of soul." Since intimacy is achieved through the development of an inner life, an absence of intimacy results from the devaluation of the inner life.

In this instance, intimacy does not refer to sexual intercourse or social discourse but to the knowledge and understanding of the deepest nature of things and their connection to one another. It is the intimacy that comes from truth and genuineness.

An absence of intimacy is reflected in virtually every problem plaguing society today. We pursue worldly gratifications over spiritual advancement and are preoccupied with the physical world, seeking wholeness from it rather than from within ourselves. An absence of intimacy is epitomized by commercialization and competition.

Commercialization encourages excessive attachments to the phenomena of celebrity and image, whether deified or vilified; acquisitionism through crass consumerism; superficial stimulations such as movies, sports, computers, etc.; and competition over cooperation. The more you have, the better off you are is the mantra of a commercialized society. Materialism, once considered a dirty word, is now glorified.

Competition thrives in any economically driven culture in which the exclusivity and superiority of individual achievement and self-promotion are valued over the inclusivity and equality of individual uniqueness and achievement as they contribute to the family and larger community. The primary goal in a competitive environment is to overcome individual powerlessness and anonymity. When the focus is on the development and protection of the individual independent of the community rather than as an indivisible part of it, family and community along with public service suffers.

This competitive focus leads to a type of narcissistic individualism that values instant gratification and results regardless of the consequences. The extent to which we have power over our own lives and the lives of others determines our self-worth

Introduction: The History Behind the Myths

and represents a superficial connection to ourselves rather than an authentic one. It also creates an irrational need to protect individual autonomy, resulting in the diminishment of a compassionate point of view and simple common sense. Manipulation and coercion become a normal part of human interactions, and we become dependent on creating adversity rather than attempting solutions in order to serve the competitive viewpoint.

Taken to this level, competition perpetuates the absence of intimacy in society. It is present in all aspects of our lives, whether at work or at play, and affects our relationships with others. Our physical, mental, and spiritual development and well-being, income, possessions, image, and experiences all become areas of gamesmanship. When on vacation, we compete with one another to stay in the best hotels, eat the best meals, and have the best sightseeing experiences, believing that we can be physically, mentally, and spiritually restored by these experiences. We even have a classic song that celebrates the competitive edge titled "Anything You Can Do I Can Do Better" by composer Irving Berlin.

The price paid for an absence of intimacy is a plethora of societal ills, including the decline of family, tradition, and morality and a rise in social conflict evidenced by repression, fanaticism, and corruption. A lack of intimacy results in a lack of concern for the greater good and contributes to

6 MYTHS ABOUT ALTERNATIVE MEDICINE

the breakdown of community. It has also led to an over-reliance on science and technology to provide answers to all our questions and the creation of an anesthetizing mass media.

Although societal problems are often compartmentalized and viewed as separate from one another in cause and effect, they are all connected to the same intimate void in our lives and are merely symptoms, not the cause, of our predicament.

A superficial connection to ourselves results in a loss of identity for the individual. Loss of identity turned inward becomes depression, and loss of identity turned outward becomes aggression and violence, which are noted in record numbers today. It also breeds fanatical hero worship and cult-like reverence of celebrities or anyone in the limelight in an effort to fill the intimate void in ourselves.

In fact, our great technological achievements such as movies, television, and computers may just represent the ultimate in convenience—an approximation of intimacy without our actually having to experience it face to face or give anything in return.

In a highly secular culture, faith in public and private institutions diminishes, transience becomes a form of stability, and kindness is mistaken for weakness. This leads to an overall loss of civility in society, cutting a swath across all social and economic strata. The absence of intimacy and the devaluation of the inner life generates detachment and apathy in the health care process and is at the

Introduction: The History Behind the Myths

heart of technology, the foundation for modern conventional medical practice.

The problem is that external preoccupations and gratifications never satisfy the spiritual need for wholeness. The hunger remains and becomes more urgent in its desire to satiate itself, growing with our increasing detachment from nature and becoming addictive without our even noticing it. Competition reinforces this need when marketing messages constantly tell us that we must have a product or service in order to lead happy, productive lives.

Trying to fill the intimate void in this way is like trying to pour water into a glass with a big hole in the bottom. A chronically unsatiated need results in chronic physical, emotional, and spiritual distress.

The consciousness movement of the 1960s, in all its wildness, attempted to initiate a return to intimacy through the advocation of peace, love, and a reconnection with nature. New concepts of medical treatment that were influenced by Eastern philosophies gained widespread recognition and were termed "bodymind medicine."

Bodymind medicine was born out of the realization that it is impossible to separate the physical from mental. Physical symptoms have mental implications, and mental symptoms have physical ones. Although the acute, killer diseases of the nineteenth and early twentieth centuries required fast-acting, invasive medical therapies, the chronic illnesses of today require the slow-acting, noninvasiveness of the bodymind approach.

A holistic approach toward health was initially the object of derision by the medical establishment. But the revolutionaries of the '60s are now the establishment and primary consumers in the new century. This shift in the ruling class and its purchasing power has allowed the concept of an integrated medicine, conventional and alternative medicine together, to emerge as an accepted approach to health. As almost one-half of our entire population faces the prospect of aging, alternative medicine is gaining widespread support and approval.

In this way, we are really returning to the original roots of medicine. Instead of a traditionally spiritual perspective on health being applied to an emerging secular science, as was true at the beginning of our medical journey, our traditionally secular and scientific perspective is now being applied to a re-emerging spirituality. This transition also signals the return of the sacred feminine and a more balanced point of view, shifting away from one of patriarchal dominance.

The acknowledgment of a bodymind connection is certainly a step in a positive direction, giving us a wider perspective on the process of healing. Without the inclusion of spirit and divine providence in the equation, however, the healing process is still incomplete. Only when we are able to regard this important aspect of health as an inseparable part of

Introduction: The History Behind the Myths

the journey will emergence from our self-imposed, spiritual Dark Ages be possible. Naturalist John Muir said that we are more *on* the world than *in* the world. The pendulum has begun to swing in the other direction.

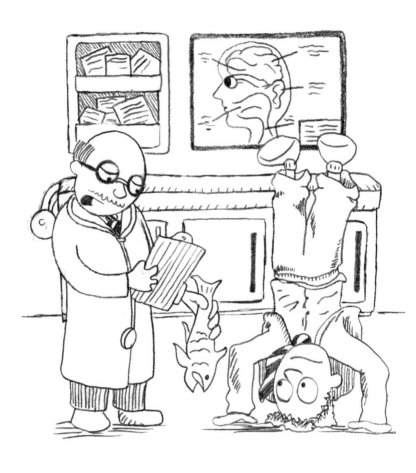
"Okay, now rub this fish all over your body."

MYTH 1

The Healer
Always Knows Best

You don't need to be helped any longer.
You've always had the power . . .

WIZARD OF OZ

From the time we are born, we are led to believe
that total deference and compliance to the opinions
of health care providers is the key to being a "good
patient." It should come as no surprise that this lifetime conditioning causes us to approach alternative
medicine in similar ways.

We continue to be "good patients" out of fear,
intimidation, and habit: fear of the unknown when
confronted with a condition over which we feel
we have no control, intimidation by a system that
insists on being in charge of our care, and the habit

of performing this role since birth. A passive, sub-missive approach to health care implies that we do not know what we need to be well and results in the myth that the healer always knows best, one that many alternative providers continue to encourage.

A belief in this myth encourages complacency on the part of the consumer, preventing us from get-ting the best care—alternative or conventional. It also prompts a desperation for answers when illness strikes, feeding a billion-dollar self-help industry in publishing, motivational speaking, and workshops.

We are encouraged to perform this role by every aspect of our society, but it is not a true reflection of our individual or collective power in the healing process. We know much more about what ails us and what we need to heal than we might possibly imagine or any medical establishment would have us believe. This does not mean, however, that we do not need anyone to help us along the way.

To be open to the thoughts, ideas, and abilities of others is a critical part of the healing process. Elemental to self-empowerment is the ability to be interdependent with those who share the same goals. Interdependence means that you have the ability to depend on others when circumstances warrant but can depend on yourself when they do not.

Healers can jumpstart the healing process with an appropriate intervention or point you in the right direction if you have veered off course. If they are particularly advanced in their respective practices

Myth One: The Healer Always Knows Best

and their hearts and minds are in the right place, healers sometimes have the ability to transmit powerful knowledge. Even so, they are only facilitators, helping you to connect with your own healing capacity.

Alternative providers who are clear about their role will tell you that you have the power to realize everything you need to heal yourself. Guidance from any healer in the form of interventions, medicines, or advice is only just that—guidance. It is not gospel or law but an instrument you can use to activate your body's natural wisdom to heal itself, even if the provider's hands appear to be doing all the work.

The value of a healer's guidance rests with your willingness to take the information that is offered and make it your own, integrating it into your personal understanding, experience, and truth. It is only as effective as your ability to apply it to your life.

Patience, discipline, and a strong desire to be empowered in the health care process are required to access and utilize the knowledge of others in order to facilitate healing in yourself. You can develop this power on your own instead of relying on the power of others.

Unwavering deference to the opinions of others or a fixation upon others to solve your problems is not the key to true healing. *Learning to listen to yourself is the key to true healing, and there is simply no shortcut to this process.* Healers do not always know what is best for you, but you do and always have, even with something as complicated as what it takes for you to be well.

Gurus

Especially popular in our society today, gurus are really just another type of healer. They are healers of the spirit, but their guidance also impacts body and mind in the holistic tradition of alternative medicine. Gurus typically have an understanding that goes beyond mere instruction in a spiritual practice or the articulation of moral lessons.

Gurus are not only Buddhist monks and turbaned Hindus but anyone who affects profound change in a person's life such as a teacher, parent, neighbor, friend, pastor, rabbi, or other spiritual advisor. The Buddhist definition of a guru is a "spiritual friend."

Gurus in other cultures are regarded differently from gurus in our culture. Although respected and treated deferentially, they are not worshiped to the exclusion of oneself. In our culture, gurus become celebrities who are transformed into godlike beings. Students often lose their identities in their reverence for a guru.

Losing your identity to a guru or any teacher points to the absence of an intimate connection to yourself rather than a genuine search for answers. It suggests that you have become intoxicated with the

Myth One: The Healer Always Knows Best

messenger instead of realizing the power his message can help you discover within yourself.

Genuine gurus usually do not claim to be gurus or especially enlightened in any way. They possess great humility and teach in the best way—by demonstration. In accordance with ancient wisdom traditions, true gurus do not encourage followers or charge money for their services. A Hindu master once said, "Gurus come to bestow and not to receive. The Guru never accepts a penny from anybody. If he does, he is not a Guru but only a beggar."

Beware the false prophet—he is in every corner to sway you from your path.

Develop Personal Health Care Power

Hippocrates, the fifth-century B.C. Greek physician who is considered to be the father of modern medicine, wrote, "the natural forces within us are the true healers of disease." If these forces are within us, we can activate and learn to use them for the purposes of understanding our own condition and knowing what to do to resolve it.

You can achieve this goal by developing personal health care power, which will also help you to address the other myths outlined in this book. To put a famous Presidential phrase in another context—"Ask not what health care can do for you; ask what you can do for your health care."

6 MYTHS ABOUT ALTERNATIVE MEDICINE

Personal health care power allows you to take responsibility for your physical, emotional, and spiritual well-being and signifies a willingness to embark on an inner journey that provides deeper meaning to the experience of health. It is an internal power that is manifested externally and suggests a deep, authentic knowledge of oneself.

Developing personal health care power is important because it:

- places you in charge of your health with the understanding that no one is more committed to your best interests than you

- allows you to take responsibility for your welfare and stop looking for others to fix or save you

- provides you with the opportunity to own past, present, and future actions

- unveils the underlying causes of your condition

- helps you to find your true nature, an integral part of the healing process

- reconnects you with nature, within which lies the ultimate cure

Knowledge is at the heart of the development of personal health care power. Unfortunately, our educational system offers little support or encouragement

Myth One: The Healer Always Knows Best

for developing this potential. In primary and secondary schools, health education consists of physical and sex education along with competitive sports. It excludes critical issues such as nutrition, stress management, mental and environmental health, and responsible health consumerism.

If we were taught to develop our health potential with the same seriousness and depth with which we are taught other subjects in our educational system, there would be less of a need to devote a chapter in any book to developing personal health care power.

The development of personal health care power involves knowing yourself, knowing the medicine you are using, and having faith in the process of healing. There are three steps you can take to develop personal health care power, which will help you to accomplish these goals. They are:

- assume an active role

- develop an inner life

- surrender to the experience

Assume an Active Role

You cannot become empowered in the health care process and get the most from any medicine unless you are willing to assume an active role in it. In my book *Is Your Health Care Killing You? 12 Ways to Survive Our Fractured Health Care System*, I suggest

6 MYTHS ABOUT ALTERNATIVE MEDICINE

that one way to do this is to begin to view yourself as a *consumer* rather than a *patient*. This minor change in terminology may seem insignificant on the surface but is profound in practice.

The role of patient signifies the complacency of the past and suggests that you are more a bystander than an equal participant in the health care process. The role of consumer signifies empowerment and a responsibility to investigate, examine, question, choose, reject, and discontinue any health service. It implies that you know what you want and can take the appropriate action to get it. Assuming this role is the first step toward developing personal health care power.

When you relinquish the traditionally passive role of patient for the activist role of consumer who participates fully in the health care process, you are able to make informed decisions and choices about your care, exercising common sense and sound judgment every step of the way. This can be as simple as deciding when to take an herb or as complex as deciding which treatment to use for a life-threatening condition.

You benefit from being able to make even the smallest choices on your own about your care. Research confirmed this when it found health benefits for elderly patients who chose their own appointment times for medical visits.

Assuming an active role takes many forms. It demands that you have positive, productive

Myth One: The Healer Always Knows Best

relationships in place with alternative providers, family, and friends in preparation for any health circumstance. An active role means choosing the right alternative providers for the right circumstance and developing collaborative partnerships with them. It also points to a willingness to raise any issue with a provider that concerns you or end a relationship with one that no longer works for you.

An active role necessitates that you investigate your condition and its underlying causes, gather all health information at your disposal, educate yourself about established and alternative treatment options, use alternative remedies responsibly, and consult with people whose opinions you trust. It involves a willingness to examine and resolve unhealthy issues, develop positive self-care habits, walk the spiritual talk, and engage in alternative medicine with as pure intentions as possible.

Assuming an active role requires knowledge of your health care rights and an ability to defend them if necessary. It also includes adequate preparation for medical emergencies. An active role also involves changing your outward focus to an inward one.

Develop an Inner Life

Healing is within everyone's grasp. When you develop personal health care power, you recognize that this capacity lies within yourself. Understanding that your body has the natural ability to heal itself is a significant step toward realizing true healing. Although there are people who will tell you that they have the answers to your problems, the truth is that no person or external intervention can do this for you. Once you are open to this possibility, many things will begin to happen.

All physical illness has an emotional and spiritual basis. We live on a biological level, several floors removed from the spirit world, where we are outwardly directed to time, space, and physical pleasures. Immersed in the physical world, predisposed by our humanness and cultural values, and as a consequence of the natural maturation process, we forget how to access our spiritual natures, which hold many answers for us.

This wisdom serves as a guide to both what is helpful and what is harmful for healing. It leads to greater meaning in life experience and continues after death. Although we often regard spiritual connectedness or intuition as a sign of weakness, fraud, or even pathology, many spiritually advanced societies regard it as a sign of supreme intelligence and superiority.

This higher source of knowledge is known by many names: intuition; instinct; heart; consciousness; psyche; psi; higher self; higher power; sixth sense; holy spirit; third eye; inner or infinite self, wisdom, voice, guidance, knowing, splendor, and light; clairvoyance; love; luminosity; creator or creative part

Myth One: The Healer Always Knows Best

of the universe; great spirit; divine force, presence, power, and will; *Tao*; and all names for God.

As anyone who is close to a pet knows, animals possess a high degree of intuitive ability. An English biologist found that pets communicate telepathically with their owners through the use of "morphic fields" and, as such, can instinctively tell when their owners are about to return home before they arrive. People with special needs have received health benefits from participation in therapeutic programs such as horseback riding and swimming with dolphins. If animal intuitiveness is good for us, then surely our own intuitiveness is good for us too.

Although we experience occasional moments of intuitiveness through our personal interactions, we lose general recognition of it as adults. Intuition tends to be more active in the beginning and ending stages of life but gets bogged down in the middle when our egos assume control. Our reliance on machines for communication and the mass media for information reduces these experiences even further. Like any part of the body that is unused for an extended period of time, our intuition can atrophy to the point at which we barely remember that it existed at all.

Some people never lose the ability to access this higher source of knowledge easily and spontaneously, but most of us can only realize it through many years of cultivation and practice. Some people develop it through methods such as breathwork,

6 MYTHS ABOUT ALTERNATIVE MEDICINE

fasting, and meditation. Connecting with your intuitive self can also involve reflection, contemplation, or finding serenity in some form of sanctuary.

Cultural pursuits, such as an appreciation of art or music, nurture our connection to the creative part of the universe. Alternative techniques such as guided imagery and hypnosis can open doors to deeper insight and awareness. Native Americans believe that wisdom is available in both dreams and illness and use sweat lodge ceremonies and vision quests to access it. Dreams have also been known to hint at future events such as on-coming illness.

This inherent power emerges in the imagination, in nature, or through the survival of an unexplainable tragedy. It is often discovered in an atmosphere of insecurity and doubt because this is the state of mind most open to exploring and accepting ideas that are beyond our immediate awareness and experience. At the very least, connecting with your higher self is about paying attention to the constant messages from the outside world that are delivered to you in small and sometimes very subtle ways.

Silence is the key to the development of an inner life. It must be experienced on a regular basis and with an inward focus rather than an outward one. Listening to your inner voice answers your questions and reveals the underlying nature of your problems on every level—physically, emotionally, and spiritually. When you activate your inner voice, you encourage the development of your natural psychic

Myth One: The Healer Always Knows Best

ability and strengthen your connection to the creative part of the universe.

The development of an inner life will automatically change your outer life. Inner wisdom always occurs in the presence of love, not anger, resentment, or fear.

Many of us learn to compensate for a lack of inner wisdom with constant analysis, careful planning, and methodical preparation. In fact, you could say we have a national obsession with these pursuits through the mistaken belief that we can control everything that happens to us. But precautions like these only work when life is going well. They become quickly ineffectual in the presence of adversity that we believe is beyond our control, at which time we are then forced to go inward and explore our inner resources to more fully understand our present circumstance.

Top 10 Ways to Develop an Inner Life

There are many ways the connection to your higher self can be cultivated and deepened, which include the following:

1. *Practice an inward-focused discipline*. There are many inward-focused disciplines, such as meditation, prayer, breathwork, trancework,

6 MYTHS ABOUT ALTERNATIVE MEDICINE

etc. Choose the discipline that most appeals to you, and practice it regularly, even if it is only a few minutes a day to start out. Your practice will change as your needs change. Be aware when this occurs and willing to go to the next level or practice to meet your changing needs.

Your practice can include some form of daily ritual or devotion, such as chanting, lighting a candle on an altar, or keeping a gratitude journal. Begin and end your day with a sense of appreciation for life's gifts and those who have contributed to your journey along the way.

2. *Fine-tune the five senses*. Pay attention to sights, sounds, smells, tastes, and touches. This encourages you to stay in the present moment. Focus on the here and now, not on what happened to you in the past or what will happen to you in the future. This will make you more aware of your current surroundings and their effect upon you.

3. *Help others*. The ability to put others before yourself cultivates *kindness* and *compassion*. Kindness and compassion, especially when directed toward difficult people, promotes *forgiveness*, another important characteristic in the development of an inner life.

Myth One: The Healer Always Knows Best

4. *Spend time in solitude.* Spend a regular period of time in absolute silence with no distractions or disturbances of any kind. The calm that results from solitude leads to greater awareness and wisdom.

5. *Spend time in nature.* Nothing activates the connection to the higher source of knowledge more than spending time in nature in such a way that you are able to notice and fully appreciate your physical surroundings.

6. *Tell the truth.* Lying, no matter how small or justified, inhibits the ability to develop a deeper connection to yourself.

7. *Look at yourself.* Be willing to look at yourself, especially when you do not like what you see. Remember that there is a serious danger of healthy self-examination turning into unhealthy self-absorption. Healthy self-examination occurs only when a situation warrants, but self-absorption is perception of self without interruption. The key is to be able to discern the difference.

8. *Take care of yourself.* Engage in healthy self-care habits by eating right, getting enough rest, and staying physically fit. The development of an inner life, which

involves the cultivation and management of psychic energy, takes both physical and mental strength and endurance.

9. *Practice one-pointedness.* Complicated, busy lifestyles that include juggling many things simultaneously at breakneck speed do not allow for the development of an inner life. Simplify your life and slow down. Nothing is as complicated as it appears to be or you make it. Savor an experience by focusing on one thing at a time.

10. *Engage in spiritual writing, reading, and association.* Recording your spiritual experiences encourages a more intimate connection to yourself. Since dreams symbolize the higher self, write them down on a regular basis. Reading about the spiritual experiences of others makes you more open to your own spiritual experiences.

    Surround yourself with like-minded individuals. Social support encourages the continuation of the inward journey. If you choose to seek the guidance of a spiritual teacher, take the time to choose one carefully, making sure that his approach is compatible with your needs, beliefs, and world view and that his teachings are substantive.

Myth One: The Healer Always Knows Best

There are a couple of intermediary techniques you can use to access your higher self. *Muscle testing* or applied kinesiology is a process of using your own muscle resistance to answer questions. There are two main ways to muscle test, but the first way works best with another person. Raise your arm shoulder-height and parallel to the ground. Ask a question, and try to keep your arm raised while the helper tries to lower your arm with both of his hands. If your arm resists lowering, the answer is yes. If your arm lowers easily, the answer is no.

This same muscle testing technique can also be used with your fingers and performed alone. Make a circle with the thumb and index finger of each hand. Place one finger circle inside the other without separating them. Ask a question, and try to separate the fingers of the outer circle with the inner one. If the fingers of the outer circle resist separation, the answer is yes. If they do not, the answer is no.

There are various *dowsing* techniques you can use to connect to a higher source of knowledge. One involves the use of a pendulum with predetermined signals for yes and no. You hold a pendulum such as a key or object over your hand or part of your body. Ask a question. Signals from the pendulum may register as tingling sensations, energetic vibrations, direct cognitions, or electric shocks. If you can dowse accurately, you can arrive at answers that are difficult to discover by any other means.

6 MYTHS ABOUT ALTERNATIVE MEDICINE

Many conventional doctors and scientists are openly critical of the view that healing comes from within. They suggest that this New Age message is irresponsible because it sets people up for failure if they cannot access this scientifically unproven resource.

First, it is doubtful that science will ever be able to fully measure or prove it. Second and most importantly, *what is irresponsible is for providers to encourage total dependency on medical intervention, then abandon people when interventions fail without helping them to develop other ways of dealing with illness and discover other avenues to healing*. Unfortunately, this is a common scenario in the practice of conventional medicine.

You can seek and heed the opinions of others until the end of time, but if you want to advance the healing process to any significant degree, you must begin to listen to your own voice rather than the voices of others. When you feel a deeper connection to this part of yourself, you will cease to look for answers elsewhere.

The most difficult part about accessing this knowledge is believing that it exists in the first place and having faith in the guidance that it provides. But every person has access to this powerful inner resource if it is allowed to surface and develop with practice. When the powers of the psyche emerge and are integrated into your life, the power to heal becomes much more likely.

Myth One: The Healer Always Knows Best

Surrender to the Experience

The ability to surrender to an experience is best expressed by the Serenity Prayer attributed to Reinhold Niebuhr, which states, "God, give us grace to accept with serenity the things that cannot be changed, courage to change the things which should be changed, and the wisdom to distinguish the one from the other." When you are connected to your higher self through the development of an inner life, you possess the wisdom to make this very important distinction.

To surrender to an experience does not mean to give up or give in. It means to have loving trust toward an experience that is for the greater good and is a natural part of the divine order of the universe.

When you surrender, you recognize that it is not possible to fix everything or do everything perfectly, and that explanations are not always necessary. Perseverance and tenacity are desirable qualities only to the extent that you can recognize their inappropriateness in the presence of obvious signs to change directions or move on.

Surrendering to your own deepest wisdom suggests a willingness to explore and implement whatever means are available to you. To surrender to an experience is to accept what is offered with grace and gratitude without losing the ability to extend love out into the world.

6 Myths About Alternative Medicine

Eastern religious traditions create an environment in which the ability to surrender is socially and culturally acceptable. Buddhists believe that life is meant for suffering as a result of worldly attachments. Hindus believe that life is an illusion, for the real world exists after death. Muslims believe that what is done in this lifetime will affect what happens in the future.

If these were the expectations of our culture, we might be less inclined toward bitterness, anger, blame, and retaliation when difficulties occur and more inclined toward understanding the true significance of surrendering to an experience.

Surrendering to an experience involves the realization that responsibility is not synonymous with blame—a common misperception. Although personal health care power involves taking responsibility for your health, it does not mean you are to blame for your illness or the inability to change its course if it worsens. Blame produces guilt, and guilt does not promote any form of healing.

To have regrets about causing or worsening your illness is to presume that life could be any other way and nothing can be gained from the experience. Instead of feeling stigmatized by disease as though you must have done something wrong to deserve it, you can be inspired by the experience.

Taking responsibility for your health signifies a commitment to look for answers and to look within, increasing awareness and opportunities for growth.

Myth One: The Healer Always Knows Best

You can change what does not have to be but surrender to what is. To look within is to search for meaning, and to search for meaning is to discover a greater plan.

If there is a higher purpose in every life experience, then guilt or shame about being or staying ill is automatically eliminated. Surrendering to the experience promotes the understanding that illness is truly an exceptional opportunity for self-discovery and growth.

Developing personal health care power may be difficult at first because it is a role that is unfamiliar to us. Like a pair of new shoes that soften and mold into a comfortable shape with time, the discomfort does not last forever. To encourage this process, surround yourself with alternative providers and other health professionals who understand their role and welcome your participation. The benefits provided by this type of empowerment will last forever and enrich every aspect of your life.

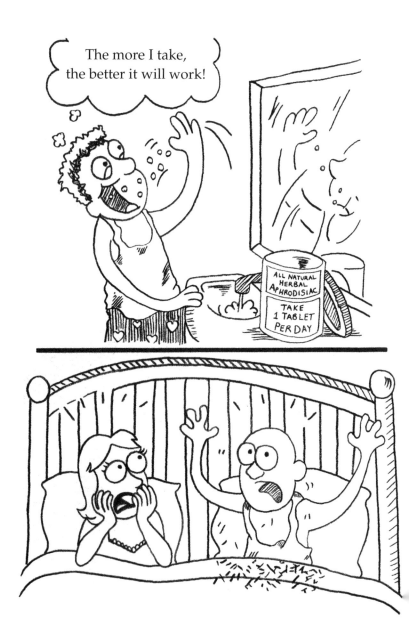

MYTH 2

It Can't Hurt You

Caveat Emptor—"Let the Buyer Beware"

The growing interest in alternative medicine has created a crowded marketplace in which various practices, therapies, treatments, and faiths hotly compete for customers and followers. Within this marketplace, we know that alternative medicine may or may not help us due to its highly individualized nature, but we also believe that alternative medicine will not harm us because of its natural and, therefore, benevolent nature.

This latter belief creates a potentially dangerous situation for the unsuspecting and uneducated consumer because alternative medicine, if not chosen carefully and used properly, *can* definitely hurt you.

Alternative medicine generates an estimated $40 billion every year in consumer spending. In any growth industry involving the potential for huge profit, there will always be legitimate along with opportunistic businesses. In alternative medicine, there are genuine healers along with snake oil salesmen and practices and therapies that are what they claim to be along with those that are not.

Alternative medicine is not extensively regulated, which is not necessarily a good or bad thing. What it does mean is that you have to be careful about what you use and whom you choose to provide it to you.

Alternative medicine is collectively and generally described as "New Age." However, some alternative practices are thousands of years old, so there is really nothing "new" about them. The media often uses this moniker disparagingly, leaving people with the impression that some measure of quackery is always involved.

Although there are certainly many suspect practices in alternative medicine, there are numerous ones that are reliable and effective. A legitimate, established alternative practice in the hands of a responsible provider is anything but quackery. But there are also providers whose only desire is to separate you from your money. Greed and narcissism

Myth Two: It Can't Hurt You

are alive and well in this business as are varying degrees of consciousness.

Buyer beware is the best rule to follow when you are navigating the alternative medicine waters. As the saying goes, "You can believe in Allah and still tie up your camel!"

Alternative Practices & Providers

There exists a common misconception that all alternative practices and providers are above reproach because the basis for alternative medicine is altruistic and because of our indoctrination as trusting conformists to any system of medicine. This is simply untrue. Blind trust toward alternative practices and providers is just as unwise as blind trust toward conventional practices and providers. Ideally, health professionals should be above practicing any type of medicine for selfish reasons, but this is a naive view since human nature is human nature regardless of the profession.

Providers of all types exist on the alternative medicine market. There are alternative providers who are properly trained and many who are not. Some providers have experience, while others are novices. There are those who are congenial and good communicators and others with the personality and warmth of Mt. Rushmore. Many alternative providers have a strong sense of ethics, but some are no better than ambulance chasers in terms of what they are willing to do to get and keep your business.

Many alternative providers embrace a holistic view in theory but not in practice. Some may try to force their views and opinions onto you without consideration for your own views and opinions; providers like these usually need you more than you need them.

There are many conventional providers who have become recent converts to alternative practice. Their conversion can signal a true appreciation for alternative medicine or it can reflect mere opportunism. Remember that providers can hurt you as much with their intent as by administering the wrong medicine.

There are many providers with what-is-colloquially-referred-to-as "ka-ching" practices. They charge excessive fees or continue to schedule regular visits when they know they cannot help you and despite a complete lack of improvement in your condition.

Practices with a spiritual focus are sometimes reduced to a commodity to be bought and sold. Be wary of anyone who uses spirituality to make money or to glorify themselves. Although the words *prophet* and *profit* are ironically pronounced the same way, in alternative medicine and especially spiritually oriented practices, *profit* is supposed to refer to the profit of the receiver, not the giver.

Many people become alternative providers simply because of their own profound healing

Myth Two: It Can't Hurt You

experiences with alternative medicine. Although firsthand experience is an asset for any alternative provider, it ensures neither competency nor success. Just because a provider is able to heal himself does not necessarily mean that he can facilitate healing in others. It is up to you to determine the extent of a provider's skill and whether his self-healing experience is an asset or a liability.

In most cases, alternative medicine is only dangerous in the hands of an unqualified or irresponsible provider. There are also those who, consciously or unconsciously, prey on medically vulnerable people.

Life-threatening and chronic illnesses such as cancer, AIDS, Alzheimer's disease, and arthritis seem to attract the most opportunities for fraud and misrepresentation because what conventional medicine can do for the people that suffer from these illnesses is severely limited. Many of these people are desperate for answers, no matter how unreasonable or ridiculous they might be. If you are in this situation, you must scrutinize alternative practices and providers carefully, employing the same caution you would use to purchase any product or service.

Bad things can happen when you put yourself in the wrong hands. One young man who was taking medication for a diagnosed mental disorder was persuaded by an alternative provider to stop taking his medication and rely solely on the provider's methods. Shortly afterward, the young man became suicidal and shot himself in the stomach. A woman with chronic, severe flu symptoms was encouraged by an acupuncturist to avoid conventional treatment. When she was finally admitted to a hospital, she was within days of dying from an undetected inflammatory disease. Although clearly worst case scenarios, experiences like these can and do happen.

Western ingenuity is capable of developing new alternative practices that are effective and beneficial, but it is also easy for those with little or no value to enter and thrive undetected in the alternative marketplace. As an educated and informed consumer, you can easily learn what to look for and what to avoid in alternative medicine. Of the latter, there are many ways to discern disreputable alternative medicine practices and providers.

Top 10 New Age Busters

You might want to avoid an alternative practice or provider if:

1. *Unrealistic claims are made about attainable results.* This includes references to products as the "perfect remedy," "miracle cure," and "ancient remedy or cure" and representations of "quick or easy results" and "a scientific breakthrough" with undocumented case histories and personal

Myth Two: It Can't Hurt You

testimonials. This caveat also pertains to providers who allege that only *their* practice, view, or path to healing will help you.

Unrealistic claims abound in alternative medicine. If an alternative medicine practice sounds too easy or too good to be true, it probably is. Headaches may be relieved by stress management techniques, but can you really be guided to "freedom, health, abundance and the spontaneous fulfillment of all your desires" in one weekend workshop, as one New Age brochure implied?

It is easy to fall prey to unrealistic claims when you are desperate for answers that conventional medicine does not possess, but there are also health conditions that are clearly better addressed by alternative rather than conventional medicine. The key is to be able to ascertain the difference between these two situations.

2. *The practice or provider is represented as the source of healing rather than a facilitator of healing.* This includes any provider who discourages your participation in the healing process, dismisses your beliefs and opinions, and places a greater value on his needs than on your own.

We seem to be stuck in the mistaken belief that an external intervener or intervention is the source of true healing and a conduit to the ultimate physical cure, as outlined in the previous chapter. You should be suspect of any provider who claims that only he or his practice has this power. If this claim is made to you, be willing to openly question it. Alternative medicine providers only facilitate and encourage the healing process, which comes from within.

Avoid providers who have a god-complex or those who need to focus an inordinate amount of attention on themselves.

3. *Intolerance for your limitations or an inability to change is part of a practice or provider's viewpoint.* This includes shaming or forcing you to do things against your will or beliefs in the name of healing.

Some alternative providers may be intolerant of your inability to comply with their wishes or to initiate a change in lifestyle or other aspect of your life. Sometimes, their expectations are justified, but sometimes, they are not. Their intolerance may reflect frustration because

Myth Two: It Can't Hurt You

they know that what they want you to do will help you. It can also point to a selfish need for control. Be wary of absolutism in the use of alternative medicine, often characterized by the use of the words "always" and "never."

The basis for alternative medicine is individual freedom and choice with respect for a person's need to take action and initiate change when he is ready for it. It is an important part of any provider's job to exercise tolerance and patience, but he can support you and encourage change at the same time by helping you to take smaller steps. Intolerance from a health provider does nothing more than create unnecessary pressure and stress, interfering with the healing process and hurting you more than helping you.

4. *The excessive or exclusive use of one remedy is used to achieve a "cure."* Singular viewpoints such as this ignore the potential of other remedies to further the cause of healing and the appropriateness of utilizing different remedies for different stages of healing. This caveat also applies to providers who diagnose a particular health condition excessively or exclusively

despite differences in symptoms or circumstances.

Sometimes, a single remedy will resolve a minor health condition without further need for intervention. Serious health conditions usually require more. Since alternative medicine is generally based on the belief that different remedies and interventions are required for different levels of healing, the exclusive use of one remedy is completely contrary to that belief.

Some alternative providers become fond of a particular diagnosis. Popular diagnoses in alternative medicine in recent years include parasite infestation, leaky gut syndrome, and chronic fatigue syndrome. Popular diagnoses have long existed in conventional medicine. For example, hypoglycemia, or low blood sugar, was widely diagnosed in the 1970s.

An illness can certainly cycle in and out, causing many people to contract it at the same time. But providers can also overdiagnose an illness because there is so much pressure on them to come up with answers. Success also brings about complacency. When a treatment resolves a condition, the provider may be inclined

Myth Two: It Can't Hurt You

to administer it to anyone with similar symptoms without proper investigation.

5. *The practice has a superficial approach to health care.* A superficial approach to health care involves symptomatic treatment without interest in or consideration for the underlying causes of illness—physical, mental, and spiritual. It also applies to alternative practices that require the adoption, promotion, or purchase of superficial accouterments or accessories in order for the treatment to be successful.

   Many alternative providers limit treatment to the alleviation of symptoms because this represents the Western view of cure. This is contrary to the holistic point of view and purpose of alternative medicine to advance the cause of true healing. Providers whose primary objective is symptom resolution are not practicing alternative medicine, and you should challenge such superficial views. Providers should be willing and able to delve deeper into the underlying causes of illness and be both knowledgeable and comfortable discussing all aspects of your health.

   An accessory-intensive approach to medicine is also part of the Western view. As

such, alternative practices employ all sorts of
material paraphernalia. Meditation practice
includes the use of beads, chant books,
chimes, bowls, incense, zafus, and zabutons
(pillows). Drums, headdresses, and rattles
are part of shamanic healing. Aromatherapy
requires pottery or electric machines to
release and disperse essential oils, and audio
tapes are used in guided imagery.

Objects such as those listed above are
helpful tools, but the success of alternative
treatment does not depend on their use.
In spiritual practices, material aids are
usually given to students free of charge
or in exchange for a donation based on
your ability to pay. Providers should never
charge clients more than their actual cost for
this merchandise.

6. *Exorbitant fees are charged for products or
services regardless of your financial status,
or advance payment is required.* Alternative
providers whose services are only available
to those who can afford them are engaging
in elitist medicine, which signals greater
concern for their personal profit than your
healing. Paying in advance for a product
or service you have not received is never
appropriate. Demands for advance payment

Myth Two: It Can't Hurt You

frequently follow bogus warnings of "limited availability."

Money is a polarizing issue in alternative medicine because it is becoming more and more expensive to use and many people are getting rich from it. But alternative medicine is based on egalitarian principles, which advocate equal treatment for people regardless of sex, race, age, education, or economic status and the social responsibility of the haves providing for the have-nots. As such, it should be available to anyone who needs it.

Elitism has no place in health care. Although the original intent of health insurance was to level the economic playing field between the haves and the have-nots, alternative medicine generally falls outside of those parameters. If an alternative practice is too costly, ask for a discount or sliding fee scale based on your ability to pay.

7. *The use of conventional medicine is discouraged during any part of the healing process, especially in life-threatening conditions.*

In life threatening or potential life-threatening conditions, this caveat is simply

6 MYTHS ABOUT ALTERNATIVE MEDICINE

non-negotiable. No matter how much your provider is convinced that alternative medicine will resolve your problem, it is irresponsible for him to encourage you to discontinue treatment with conventional medicine.

If you are pressured by a provider to discontinue conventional treatment and have reservations about doing it, get a second opinion. If you choose to discontinue conventional treatment on your own, you must take responsibility for the consequences. In the absence of a life-threatening situation, you can probably use alternative medicine on its own, monitoring your condition to make sure it does not deteriorate into something more serious.

8. *The extent of professional training in an alternative medicine technique consists of workshops, courses, lecture series, or symposiums lasting only a few weekends, weeks, or months.*

Due to its popularity, alternative medicine training programs and schools have cropped up all across the country. Some of them consist of only one or two weekend seminars, after which

Myth Two: It Can't Hurt You

participants hang out a shingle claiming expertise in the practice or technique. Training programs that are only a few weeks or months in length may not be much better, depending on the practice or technique. For example, 300–400 hours of training in a complex practice such as acupuncture is grossly inadequate, but the same number of hours in a bodywork technique may be sufficient.

Training in an alternative practice or technique is not the only criterion that matters. Expertise is also forecast by the experience of the provider. Alternative providers with little training and experience are more common than you might think.

9. *Spiritual enlightenment is guaranteed.*

Any alternative provider who promises spirituality as though it can be easily acquired or transferred from one person to another like a possession or an object is not connected with his own spirituality and is selling you something else.

Spirituality for sale is an abhorrent concept for all the obvious reasons. Even so, it flourishes in our culture, and we collectively spend an estimated one billion dollars every year to become spiritually enlightened. But no one can give spirituality to you because you already have it. You must simply find the means to connect with it. Spirituality is always present and can only be realized through years of dedication and hard work.

10. *No improvement in your condition is perceived within a reasonable period of time for alternative medicine.*

This raises another misconception in health care that hurts us in our use of alternative medicine. If the medicine does not produce immediate results, we believe that either it is the wrong medicine or the medicine is no good.

Alternative treatments and remedies take longer to work than conventional treatments and drugs, and symptoms of illness can sometimes worsen before improving. True healing is not a speedy process, especially in the presence of a serious health condition. If you cannot overcome this unrealistic expectation, alternative medicine will always disappoint.

Myth Two: It Can't Hurt You

Alternative Products

There are thousands of alternative medicine products on the market. Merchandise like crystals, fountains, chimes, music, clothing, jewelry, and artwork can be pleasing and harmless additions to your environment. Products with medicinal value such as alternative remedies and herbs are a different story, whether they are taken internally or used externally.

Knowledge of the nature, properties, and power of alternative remedies and herbs is essential not only for their success but also to avoid harm. There are huge variances in the same remedy or herb in quality, potency, dosage, and manufacturing process, which includes how the herbs are harvested, processed, stored, and packaged.

Like alternative therapies in general, alternative remedies and herbs are usually only harmful in the wrong hands. You must still watch out for the occasional product with harmful ingredients that manages to slip by regulators. Also, if a remedy is not applied properly with consideration for all health factors, an old problem can worsen or a new one arise where there was none before.

Adverse reactions to herbal remedies are not uncommon. Some remedies are toxic in high doses and lose their potency with prolonged use. There can be negative interactions between alternative remedies

6 MYTHS ABOUT ALTERNATIVE MEDICINE

and other herbs or drugs. Adverse reactions can manifest physically, emotionally, and spiritually.

A well-known example of potential harm from an alternative remedy involves the herb ephedra. Ephedra, also known as the Chinese herb *Ma huang*, is a shrub-like plant found in the Asian desert. The root of this plant was originally used to reduce sweating and was later used for bronchial problems such as asthma. It is now used as a weight loss remedy and recreational drug because it stimulates the central nervous system and increases the heart rate with an effect similar to speed.

Overuse and abuse of ephedra has serious consequences, increasing blood pressure and causing cardiac arrhythmia and even death from heart failure. Since 1993, the Food and Drug Administration (FDA) has received thousands of reports of adverse reactions (almost 1,200 adverse reactions in 2001 according to the U.S. Poison Control Centers) and 155 deaths from the use of ephedra, resulting in a nationwide ban on its sale.

You must exercise caution and educate yourself before using medicinal remedies and herbs. (See Myth 3.)

New Age Conferences & Workshops

Along with the deluge of alternative practices, products, and publications on the market, there is also a thriving business of conferences, workshops,

Myth Two: It Can't Hurt You

lectures, seminars, and travel tours on alternative medicine. This New Age circuit features many people who are regarded as leaders in the field of alternative medicine and includes instructional and experiential presentations. These events take place globally and are advertised in New Age magazines, newspapers, on the Internet, and by direct mail.

Presenters at these events are usually providers of alternative therapies and techniques who are famous for writing books about their own professional and healing experiences. Many of them are psychotherapists with expertise in the bodymind connection. There are also medical doctors, researchers, anthropologists, historians, philosophers, educators, motivational speakers, and performance artists. Many presenters have discontinued private practices and academic careers in order to lecture on the New Age circuit, making their living through lucrative speaking fees, product sales, and newsletter subscriptions.

Alternative medicine conferences and workshops are helpful in two ways: as an introduction to the basic concepts in alternative medicine and holistic healing and as an opportunity to network with people of similar interests. At large New Age events, a variety of alternative practices and therapies are represented at one time, allowing you to compare and contrast their various approaches to health and healing. Connecting with like-minded individuals is not only fertile ground for fellowship but also allows you to learn about other people's experiences with alternative medicine.

As a novice, shopping the alternative medicine marketplace and trying new techniques and therapies helps you to discover the practices that best suit your needs. Ongoing experimentation without commitment to any particular practice, however, does not promote growth because you cannot improve or excel in one technique or therapy if you are preoccupied with others at the same time. Chronic dabbling in alternative practices encourages only their superficial use, limiting a practice's ability to benefit you.

If you are looking for a deep, transformative experience, you will probably be disappointed with most large-scale New Age events because they are not designed for this purpose. Presenters tend to be the same from workshop to workshop, and much of the material offered to participants is a condensed version of their most recently published book. Presenters and retailers also use these events as an opportunity to sell merchandise, such as books, video and audio tapes, artwork, jewelry, and other New Age paraphernalia. Costs to attend New Age conferences and workshops can also be quite expensive.

New Age events sometimes include experiential workshops in which healings are conducted on a large scale. Although group healings can be positive experiences, they can also cause problems because

Myth Two: It Can't Hurt You

there is little or no opportunity for individual screening or follow-up care. For example, one participant in a well-known shamanic workshop experienced so much dizziness and disorientation from a group healing that she was unable to be physically active for two weeks. Exercise great care when attending experiential workshops.

Do not expect too much from the people who lead these events. One participant consulted the workshop facilitator about a serious problem, but reported being shunned by him for the remainder of the session, causing the participant enormous distress and limiting her ability to benefit from the workshop. After hearing a presentation by a well-known psychotherapist at a New Age conference, an audience member wrote him a long letter, making intimate disclosures and requesting a referral to someone qualified to help. The letter was never acknowledged with a response.

In many ways, the self-help industry exists only to help itself. Its very success is dependent on your lack of faith in your own wisdom and your belief that their products and services have the answers to your problems.

Most people, no matter how famous they are or how many followers they possess, can only speak with authority about their own experiences and are not experts on yours. You should not revere anyone to the exclusion of yourself or your own unique path to healing. Losing yourself in the identity of

6 Myths About Alternative Medicine

any teacher will not ultimately further your own cause. You can still benefit from the message, however, without becoming attached to the messenger. (See Myth 1.)

Big egos, platitudes, and self-interest all thrive on the New Age conference and workshop circuit. Any person who claims knowledge and insight into the secrets of the universe or claims to know more about you than you do warrants a closer look. An ability to distinguish true knowledge and insight from a well-developed talent for public speaking and self-promotion is helpful in separating the genuine from the phoney on the New Age circuit. The real danger in alternative medicine occurs when *self-promotion cloaked as altruism becomes false advertising, and people who are desperate for answers are unable to recognize the difference.*

Although New Age events are certainly fun and educational, they can also be more about entertainment and retail sales than true healing or transformation. With this admonition in mind, you can participate in them and enjoy their unique and inspiring atmosphere.

Alternative medicine practices, providers, and products of all types and qualities abound in the New Age marketplace. Using alternative medicine safely is about exercising simple common sense and

Myth Two: It Can't Hurt You

sound judgment, doing your homework, asking the right questions, finding good people to help you, and not being afraid of moving on if the situation warrants. If you are willing to assume these responsibilities, you will save time and money and significantly reduce your chances of being hurt.

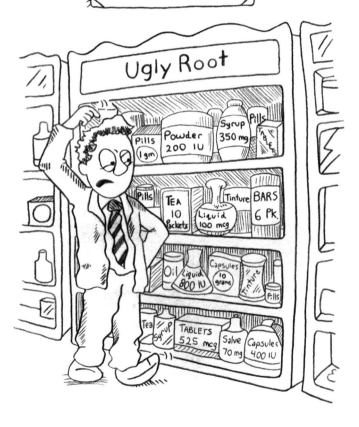

MYTH 3

All Remedies Are
Created Equal

*There are some remedies worse
than the disease.*

PUBLILIUS SYRUS

All alternative medicine remedies are not created
equal. The process by which they are made and the
forms that they take can differ greatly. There are also
variances in the circumstances under which they are
best administered. The quality of the herb, the manufacturing process, and how you use it determine
the effectiveness of an alternative remedy.

For the most part, you get what you pay for with
alternative remedies. If the remedy is inexpensive,
the quality will generally be poor. The best remedies
are usually, but not always, the most expensive ones.

Everyone has jumped on the herbal band-
wagon. Consumer demand is high, so thousands

of alternative products have flooded the market. There are more choices of remedies and herbs than ever before, making them more accessible to us but also making the selection process more arduous.

While most herbs are not inherently dangerous, they can become so in the wrong hands. In order to use them properly, you must learn as much about them as possible.

What & Where

Alternative remedies include a variety of products possessing medicinal value: nutritional supplements, Western and Eastern herbs, essential oils, flower essences, homeopathic medicines, and other remedies. They come in a variety of forms: creams, oils, gels, powders, granules, liquids, extracts, tinctures, tonics, tablets, capsules, gelcaps, syrups, liniments, salves, dermal patches, sprays, soups, teas, and herbs in their natural state.

Herbal formulas can consist of only one part or several parts of a plant and can be made from the leaf, root, flower, seeds, bark, stems, or fruit. Some remedies are comprised of only one herb; others combine several herbs together in the same formula. The anthology of Western herbs is not considered as complete as Eastern herbs, so many people prefer to use them together.

Alternative remedies, herbs, and supplements are found not only in natural food and herb stores but in

Myth Three: All Remedies Are Created Equal

almost every supermarket, pharmacy, discount chain store, on the Internet, by mail-order catalog, in television and radio infomercials, plant nurseries, and many other places. Where you buy remedies is important because of variances in the quality of products and variances in the business practices of the establishments that sell them. If you are unhappy with an alternative remedy, reputable retailers will allow you to return unused portions for a full refund.

A Complex Process

What makes choosing an herbal remedy so complex is that more than one remedy often addresses the same complaint, a variety of herbal remedies are sometimes required to address different levels of the same underlying cause, different remedies may be needed for different seasons of the year, and a remedy or dosage that works for one person may not work in the same way for another person. Alternative remedies can be toxic in higher doses, compromised when combined with other herbs or conventional drugs, and rendered ineffective if factors such as an unhealthy lifestyle or serious illness are ignored. It is also very easy to misuse an herb or a remedy. The difficulty does not end here.

Once you decide upon a particular remedy or herb, there are usually ten to twenty versions of the same herb in various forms and combinations. The action of a single herb differs from the action of a combination of herbs. A formula that combines herbs together acquires characteristics and properties all its own.

Remedies and herbs are also formulated in a wide variety of strengths, usually described in milligrams or grams. One strength may be too much for your ailment but another may be too little to have any effect at all.

Take the herb echinacea. There are at least 100 different alternative medicine remedies that contain the herb echinacea. Echinacea is found in homeopathic cold and flu remedies, herbal cold and flu remedies, allergy remedies, immune strengthening remedies, and on its own in various tinctures and capsules. It is combined with golden seal, bayberry, vitamin C, oregon grape, *astragalus*, and *reiski*. Echinacea is also found in various cough syrups with other herbs such as elderberry. Super echinacea formulas include the root juice, seed, leaf juice, and flower juice. Other products contain the root alone; root and leaf; stem, leaf, and flower; root, flower, and seed; and standardized extract and powder. Echinacea remedies vary in strength from less than 100 milligrams to more than one gram of the herb.

How They Differ

Herb quality and potency vary greatly in terms of how the herbs are grown, harvested, processed, stored, and packaged. Careful consideration of quality and

Myth Three: All Remedies Are Created Equal

potency is as important as choosing the right herb in the first place. To ensure the best quality, purchase reputable, brand name remedies and herbs from reputable retailers. Potency is a more complicated measurement. The amount of an herb contained in a formula is only one measure of the potency of an alternative remedy. Contrary to popular belief, *greater strength does not necessarily mean greater potency.*

Standardized formulas are remedies whose ingredients are analyzed to determine the percentage content of the herb and are manufactured in both liquid and solid forms. There are two basic types of standardized remedies: an active constituent extract, which concentrates one or more active constituents of the herb; and a marker extract, in which the active constituents are not known but a characteristic compound is used as a marker.

There has been a recent emphasis on developing greater consistency in and higher potency of standardized remedies. Professional herbalists take issue with this, arguing that standardized formulas cannot replace whole, nonstandardized herbs. Although an herb may contain hundreds of constituents, the standardized remedy may contain only one or two of those constituents in a highly concentrated form with effective constituents missing from the formula.

Even when all constituents are present in a standardized remedy, there is no guarantee that the herbs are aged properly or grown in optimum conditions, which, in great part, determines the herb's

6 MYTHS ABOUT ALTERNATIVE MEDICINE

strength. Critics point to inconsistencies in the manufacturing process for standardized herbs. They also believe that standardized remedies were created more to serve medical science than consumers and are supported by pharmaceutical companies, which are allowed to patent them.

In short, standardized formulas do not always ensure the highest quality and potency of the herb and are not necessarily superior to a whole, fresh, or properly aged herb that is grown in optimum conditions. There are also many herbs that are rejected by manufacturers of standardized remedies because the active constituents of the herb do not meet industry standards. These rejected herbs sometimes end up in the hands of manufacturers who add other ingredients to them and then label them standardized.

In general, the fresher the herb, the better the herbal remedy. Herbs should be chosen in the following order: whole fresh herbs, dried herbs, liquid tinctures, and freeze-dried herbs.

Whole fresh herbs are always preferable to all other choices. Dried herbs should be stored properly and protected from environmental elements. Liquid tinctures can be made with fresh or dried herbs and are usually preserved in an alcohol base. For people who are alcohol-sensitive, liquid tinctures are also preserved in a glycerin base. Freeze-dried herbs are fresh plants that are immediately frozen. Herbs that are dried naturally or exposed to oxidation are the least desirable choice.

Myth Three: All Remedies Are Created Equal

Herb potency is destroyed by heat, bacteria, air, and light. Herbs should be stored in tightly sealed jars or containers that are dark-colored and kept in a cool, dark location away from heat or light. Generally speaking, the fresher the herb, the quicker the spoilage.

Whole, uncut herbs last longer than broken or crushed herbs, usually from one to two years. Herbs with a high degree of oil will spoil quicker than those without oil. On the other hand, some herbs that are harvested from barks can actually improve with age.

Dried herbs last the longest, but they also have to be broken down in some way to release their properties. Dried herb capsules last longer than dried bulk herbs because capsules provide a degree of protection from destructive environmental elements. Powders last a few months to a couple of years, depending on how they are stored. Oils and salves can last for several years if they are preserved and stored properly. Herbs that have lost their medicinal potency can be used externally for beauty treatments and baths.

Apart from the fresh whole herb, available forms of alternative remedies, herbs, and supplements include the following:

Capsule

Capsules are best for taking strong herbs individually or in formulas and are an alternative to teas.

6 Myths About Alternative Medicine

Those made of animal or vegetable gelatins are generally more easily assimilated into the body than more concentrated tablets and pills. Capsules containing herbal powders need to be checked for adulteration.

Tablet or Pill

Tablets or pills are usually taken for chronic illnesses and have the advantage over capsules of being entirely herbal since the capsules themselves can be made of animal gelatin. But tablets can be difficult to digest and assimilate and can also contain a binding agent, which holds the herbs together. Binding agents include guar gum, acacia bark, slippery elm, dicalcium phosphate, and magnesium sterate. Chinese pills tend to have fewer binding agents than pills made using the standard methods.

Tablets are typically made from a heating process, which can alter or damage the properties of the herb. There are reportedly new methods of making tablets that avoid this outcome.

Tincture

Tinctures contain medicinal constituents of the herb that are extracted into solvents of alcohol, vinegar, or glycerine. Certain solvents work better with certain herbs in extracting the most properties from them. They have a long shelf life and are best taken in small doses. People who have a sensitivity to alcohol-based tinctures can use glycerine-based tinctures, sometimes characterized as less effective.

Myth Three: All Remedies Are Created Equal

Powder

Herbal powders can have substances added to them in order to increase their longevity or to make them cheaper. The source of the herbal powder should be checked along with its color, texture, and smell to avoid adulteration.

Tea

Medicinal teas can be made of mild or strong-tasting herbs. A tea used externally on the body is termed a wash. Be sure that packaged medicinal teas do not contain artificial colors, preservatives, or dioxin, a chemical used to bleach the tea bag.

Juice

Herbs and medicinal foods that are pulverized into a highly concentrated form of the plant or food are called juices. Remember that fresh herbs spoil very quickly. Juice should be as fresh as possible to maximize its nutritional value because it does not retain its potency for very long.

Salve

Salves are solidified oils that are combined with herbal extracts. They can also be made with alcohol or vinegar. Salves are rubbed into the skin for therapeutic purposes, usually to treat muscles, ligaments, inflammation, and bruises and to increase circulation.

Oil

Also used externally, oils are extracted from the active principles of the herb. Massage oils are either cooling and soothing or warming and stimulating. Essential oils comprise only one part of an herb so they may not be appropriate to use for certain health conditions.

Soup

Herbal soups consist of herbs cooked with meats and vegetables over a long period of time for the purposes of strengthened immunity and overall balance. Again, heat alters the properties of herbs, so cooking them at low temperatures is advisable.

Syrup

Syrups contain whole fresh or dried herbs combined with a sweetener and are used to treat throat ailments and coughs. Sweeteners can sometimes affect the properties of the syrup. Syrups should be made with natural sweeteners like molasses or honey rather than white sugar because sugar has no nutritional value and contributes to health problems. Syrups have a very short shelf life.

Suppository

Herbs combined with binding ingredients such as glycerine or cocoa butter are made into suppositories for insertion into the rectum or vagina for

Myth Three: All Remedies Are Created Equal

hormonal imbalance or other therapeutic purposes. Suppositories can be messy to use and must be kept in a cool, dry place.

Bath

A few drops of essential oil or herbs are used in baths for therapeutic purposes. They make contact with the surface of the skin and can be absorbed into the body. The general rule is that the more severe the health condition, the more frequent the herbal bath.

As you can see, there are a variety of factors to consider when selecting the right alternative remedy and dosage for medicinal purposes. This can be an exhausting process. Since there are so many variances in herbs and their use is so individualized, the generic prescription of supplements and herbs offered to the public through television shows, radio programs, and Internet websites is only a first step.

For example, many women have read about the health benefits of a popular herb arginine, which is used to improve sex drive in postmenopausal women. They rush out to buy it, automatically assuming it is right for them without further evaluation or consideration of other relevant factors. A generic prescription for an ailment is helpful in beginning your search because it narrows your

6 MYTHS ABOUT ALTERNATIVE MEDICINE

choices, but you must investigate all options and refine your selection, making sure that it is the right one for you.

Government Regulation & Manufacturer Information

There is a myth perpetuated by the conventional medical community and pharmaceutical industry that the herbal remedy and supplement market is completely unregulated. This is simply untrue.

The Food and Drug Administration requires herb and supplement manufacturers to identify the source of the plant extract (root, leaf, etc.) and concentration of the active ingredient. The federal Food, Drug, and Cosmetic Act ensures that herbal products are not adulterated. Common law of every state requires manufacturers to assure the safety of their products prior to marketing them. The U.S. Department of Agriculture has published federal standards for organic products, and many states regulate how organic foods are grown and processed, such as the California Organic Foods Act of 1990.

The Dietary Supplement Health and Education Act of 1994 (DSHEA) sets additional guidelines for manufacturers of herbs, which were recently updated. Dietary supplements are now defined as dealing with the structure or function of the body rather than the treatment of disease. This is an

Myth Three: All Remedies Are Created Equal

important distinction that allows for the continued over-the-counter distribution of herbs and supplements, which is desirable as long as we are willing to do our part to ensure their safe use.

Alternative remedies, herbs, and supplements are designed for self-use; however, herbal manufacturers do not always provide all the information that you need to make an informed choice. They do not disclose how fresh the herbs are to begin with or provide details about the manufacturing process. Manufacturers typically do not specify adverse reactions, other than to state that you should discontinue use if unusual symptoms occur. They also do not tell you about potential interactions with other herbs or drugs, which you must research on your own. It is fair to assume, however, that the more a manufacturer discloses about the product, the better the product probably is.

Manufacturers of alternative remedies and herbs and the retailers who sell them are understandably concerned about the negative effect of too much federal regulation of and control over their products. There are still those, however, who will take advantage of the public by representing a product to be something it is not. Despite governmental guidelines, alternative remedies that make false claims or contain dangerous ingredients can still exist undetected in the marketplace. More regulation is not the answer; better consumerism is.

Dangers & False Claims

Alternative remedies have faced some high profile growing pains in recent years. In addition to the herb ephedra, which was discussed in the previous chapter, manufacturing problems with L-tryptophan caused more than 30 deaths and led to its withdrawal from the market in the 1980s. Today, you can only get L-tryptophan with a prescription from a medical doctor.

In the 1990s, several natural progesterone creams arrived on the market to be used as a treatment for PMS and menopausal symptoms. Research then found that many of the creams that claimed to replace progesterone in the body actually had little or no progesterone in them at all. Recent research exposed drug interaction problems with the herb St. John's wort, and adverse outcomes have drawn attention to the extraction process used to make the herb kava kava.

In recent years, Chinese patent medicines have been found to contain additives and contaminants such as antibiotics, psychotropics, anti-inflammatories, steroids, mercury, lead, and even arsenic, which have slipped by U.S. Custom's officials. Regarding the latter three ingredients, heavy metal poisoning can produce flu-like symptoms and cause organ damage and failure. *In Bu Human*, a Chinese patent medicine used for insomnia, was found to contain a sedative similar to Thorazine.

Myth Three: All Remedies Are Created Equal

Ingredients of remedies are typically listed on package inserts and labels; however, you cannot identify them if they are omitted from inserts and labels or if they are listed in another language.

Although adverse reactions to alternative medicine remedies are rare due to their natural sources and gentle, diluted properties, they are still possible. Ginko, a popular herbal remedy used to improve mental processes by increasing blood flow to the brain and thinning the blood, can cause headaches and even hemorrhages. DHEA, an anti-aging remedy for fatigue, may cause aggressiveness and facial hair in women. Chronic use of the herb valerian can render it ineffective.

Alternative medicine remedies cannot compensate for an unhealthy lifestyle, and they are also not intended for long-term use. Chronic use of remedies and herbs can cause problems in the absence of proper evaluation and the resolution of underlying issues. Chronic use can also cause remedies to become ineffective or toxic. It is always a good idea to stop taking an herbal remedy periodically for several days and resume after the body has had an opportunity to rest from it.

To avoid the possibility of false claims, dangerous chemicals, and hazardous reactions, purchase remedies from reputable alternative providers, herbalists, health food stores, or other retailers rather than from unknown or unsolicited sources. Consult books like the Herbal Products

Association's *Botanical Safety Handbook* for a list of botanicals and their dangers. The more you know about herbal remedies, the better choices you will make.

Do not use products that are unfamiliar to you. If the claims made about a remedy cannot be verified or seem unreasonable to you, do not buy it. If you have any doubt about the legitimacy, potency, efficacy, or safety of an alternative remedy, first consult a qualified herbalist or botanical specialist.

Next, follow the recommended dose listed on the manufacturer's label, unless so prescribed by a qualified herbalist or botanical specialist. Inform your medical doctor about your use of alternative remedies, especially if you are pregnant, have medicinal allergies, or are seriously ill. Interactions are possible between conventional drugs and alternative remedies, which can alter the potency and effectiveness of either medicine and result in serious side effects.

Herbalists

Working with a qualified herbalist or botanical specialist is an invaluable aid in using alternative remedies and herbs properly and getting the most out of them. Choose an herbalist who is well trained and experienced in the use of medicinal plants and foods. Some herbalists will prescribe formulas over the phone or by email without meeting you face to

Myth Three: All Remedies Are Created Equal

face, even though there is no replacement for the personal consultation. Visual contact provides the herbalist with important information that cannot be ascertained any other way.

Good herbalists are typically found by word of mouth. You can also find herbalists through professional associations. Many herbal associations have referral lists of members, which are available to the public. Membership in a professional association, however, does not guarantee competence. You still need to investigate and evaluate an herbalist's credentials on your own.

Associations for herbalists include the following:

American Botanical Council (512) 926–4900
American Herbalists Guild (770) 751–6021
American Association of Naturopathic
    Physicians (866) 538–2267
American Horticulture Therapy Association
    (800) 634–1603
Bach Flower Essences International Education
    Program (800) 334–0843
Herb Research Foundation (303) 449–2265
World Wide Essence Society (978) 369–8454

Many alternative providers sell remedies, herbs, and supplements in their practices. They include medical doctors, chiropractors, osteopaths, acupuncturists, and naturopaths among others. Some of them possess the proper training and experience to prescribe and dispense alternative remedies, but many of them do not, choosing to stock products merely for the convenience of customers.

Health providers should only sell products to you for their actual cost. Charging more than their actual cost for a product compromises their objectivity and the quality of care that you receive. When profit is involved, how can you know whether the provider is recommending a remedy to you because you really need it or because he merely wants to make the sale?

Guidelines for Choosing & Using Alternative Remedies

1. Consult with a qualified herbalist or botanical specialist about the right remedy and dosage for your needs.

2. Determine how fresh the herbs are and how the remedy is made.

3. Check the ingredients for both source (does the remedy contain the whole herb or only some of its parts?) and concentration of the herb (how much of it is actually in the remedy?).

Myth Three: All Remedies Are Created Equal

4. Determine if the claims made by the herbal manufacturer are reasonable.

5. Find out how long a remedy should be taken.

6. Investigate the effect of the remedy on other herbs and medications you are taking.

7. Do not exceed the recommended dose.

8. Pay attention to any changes in your condition—physical, mental, and spiritual.

9. Discontinue use in the event of an adverse effect or reaction.

10. Keep your medical doctor informed about your use of alternative remedies.

In order to use alternative medicine remedies safely, responsibly, and effectively, you must be willing to educate yourself extensively about herbs and their uses. Only then can you ask the type of question that will allow you to make informed choices.

Finding the right remedy at the right time for the right circumstance is a lengthy process. Once the right remedy is found and used in the proper manner, the results can be profound.

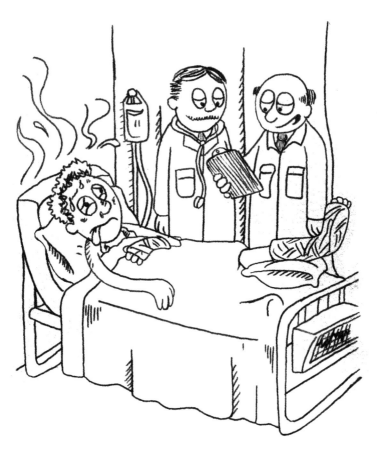

"Good news! We're releasing you because the tests say you're in perfect heallth!"

MYTH 4

You Can't Use It
Without Proof

A way of seeing is a way of not seeing.

KENNETH BURKE

A new frontier of medical science is the study of alternative medicine and its ability to enhance our natural immunity. Millions of dollars are now being allocated each year toward this type of research. For example, the budget for alternative medicine at the National Institutes of Health has risen from $2 million in 1993 to $50 million in 1999 to $105 million for 2002, $74 million of which was spent on research grants alone. Despite the dramatic increase in funds, scientific evidence on alternative medicine is still lacking.

6 Myths About Alternative Medicine

As a relatively new field of inquiry, there is considerable scepticism toward the safety and effectiveness of alternative medicine. These doubts, along with an absence of scientific validation and the possibility for exploitation, cause many critics of alternative medicine to "throw out the baby with the bath water." Academic brainwashing has led to the unfair dismissal of any alternative medicine practice or therapy that has not been thoroughly documented by science. However, there are negative aspects to any business or practice. Like everything else, alternative medicine is not all bad nor is it all good.

Not only medical scientists but also leaders in the field of alternative medicine constantly tell us that we cannot believe in the safety or effectiveness of alternative medicine unless proven so by randomized, controlled clinical trials. Certainly, no conventional provider would consider prescribing any medicine without the stamp of scientific approval. In 1998, the editors of the *Journal of the American Medical Association* (JAMA) boldly proclaimed, "until solid evidence is available that demonstrates the safety, efficacy, and effectiveness of specific alternative medicine interventions, uncritical acceptance of untested and unproven alternative medicine therapies must stop."

Skepticism overshadows trust in our society and perhaps rightly so. Our preference for the skepticism of science over the intimacy of faith is an illustration of our own spiritual impoverishment and, in

Myth Four: You Can't Use It Without Proof

the deepest sense, represents our inability to trust ourselves.

The basis for this myth is the same one described in Myth 1—an inability to trust our own judgment. This inability leads to an over-reliance on the opinions of others and makes us especially vulnerable to academic brainwashing. In a spiritually impoverished society, "prove it" is the national mantra, and nowhere is this more evident than in science and medicine.

We are more concerned with what is proven over what is logical or true, which is why science has such an intractable grip on our lives. This concern also creates a preoccupation with analysis, planning, and preparation to answer our questions and solve our problems. Science is used as a replacement for simple common sense.

A dependence on science to tell us what to do and when to do it obscures our own innate wisdom. Science says, "I don't believe without proof," but faith says, "I believe in the absence of proof." Within this dichotomy lies a serious conflict that warrants our consideration.

With respect for the important achievements advanced by science, do we really need it to tell us that joy, hope, or altruism has a positive effect on our health? To what extent is science supposed to answer *all* our questions, and do we really want to view ourselves exclusively through its lens? Would the prophets Jesus and Mohammed survive the harsh glare of scientific scrutiny today or would they also be dismissed as frauds by those who only believe in what can be quantified and measured? Is seeing really believing or are there other ways to see?

Viewpoint of Science

As outlined in the Introduction, science arose from Greek and Roman civilizations and, as a creation of man, was not always a part of our history. As such, the scientific viewpoint has its limitations regarding the ability to explain everything that happens to us and account for all phenomena.

Science is compartmentalized into numerous disciplines with little or no relationship to one another. These disciplines follow certain common procedures of investigation, analysis, and argument. Although science may focus the topic of inquiry, one academic noted that it also "creates tunnel vision and narrows our natural view" of things.

Science is based on the fragmentation of nature in which the parts are separated from the whole for the purpose of investigation. For example, science examines one part of the human body and then applies this understanding to the entire body. This fragmentation results in a detached point of view, objectifying nature and all living things that are part of it. In medicine, these fragmented, objectified living things happen to be people. Writer John

Myth Four: You Can't Use It Without Proof

Brunner said, "If there is such a phenomenon as evil, it consists in treating another human being as a thing."

The intention of science is to be objective, but this detached viewpoint also encourages a detachment from ourselves. There is no room to consider the deeper meaning of an experience. Since science values only that which it can account for, it promotes the mistaken belief that we are the masters of our destiny and anything of worth can be explained. According to science, what cannot be explained must therefore be accidental, coincidental, and ultimately insignificant.

Alternative medicine is based on the value of individual differences, but science says that a phenomenon is only significant if it occurs for the majority of people at the same time or within the confines of the study period. This is not an approach that honors or respects the value of individual experience because it is based on assembly line medicine, applying the same medicine to everyone regardless of individual needs.

If a truth does not apply to the majority of people at a given moment in time, is it then not valid for the individuals who experience that truth in the same moment in time? Does it make any sense to deny the experience of these individuals or to disallow others from trying a medicine or treatment simply because the people for whom it worked are in the minority? After all, an absence of scientific evidence is not synonymous with an absence of proof.

An over-reliance on science and the inability to trust ourselves results in an inability to trust our own experiences. For decades and despite claims from countless women, doctors insisted there was no emotional or psychological connection to female hormonal fluctuation, convincing many women that the problem was "all in their heads" and leading many of them to mistaken diagnoses of mental illness. This viewpoint seems absurd today, and this biological relationship is accepted without question by the medical establishment.

Over a decade ago, I tried to tell a sleep disorder researcher that sleep deprivation adversely affected my work performance. He denied that my experience was valid simply because there was no scientific evidence to support my claim. However, studies now show that sleep deprivation has a profound effect on the ability to function, one study suggesting that it is the equivalent of being drunk.

These examples demonstrate that science is extremely fickle, reversing its opinion repeatedly with the discovery of new studies and methods of investigation. Eggs were good for us, they were bad, and now they are good for us again. Butter is better than margarine, margarine is better than butter, and butter is better than margarine again. Soy is good for us; unless it is fermented, soy is bad for us. You must exercise every day; you must exercise three times

Myth Four: You Can't Use It Without Proof

per week for 30 minutes; you must exercise in ten minute intervals; and now you must exercise every day for one hour to be fit and to promote health. Science told us that we would be happier divorced than in unhappy marriages, but another study now claims that there is no difference between the two statuses.

Nowhere is the inconsistency of science more evident than in the study of hormonal replacement therapy (HRT) for women. Previous studies found that oral contraceptives cause breast cancer, a recent study showed that it did not, and a subsequent study showed that it did again. Research also claimed that estrogen prevents heart disease, causing millions of women to take it, but new studies found that it actually increases a woman's risk for heart attack instead of reducing it. And so on.

Science is far from being perfect or swift. The wheels of science move slowly; studies and their replication can span many years. Even after findings are replicated several times with the same results, there are always exceptions to the rule.

In experimental science, controlled studies also present ethical concerns. In order to study the effect of a particular treatment, one group of participants in the study typically receives the treatment while the control group does not. Researchers have attempted to correct this inequity by providing the treatment to the control group at the end of the study. However, if you needed a potentially effective medical treatment, would you want to wait months or even years until a study was over to receive it?

With billions of dollars in funding, science is not immune from the pressures of any business for profit. In fact, many observers believe that medical science has become irrevocably corrupt because the results of studies are often influenced by the very companies that sponsor them. Competition for research dollars, professional pressure to produce significant results, and the prestige and notoriety that accompany scientific discoveries take priority over the search for knowledge and other altruistic concerns.

Given all this, how can the skepticism and logic of science be successfully applied to the faith and mysticism that are such an integral part of alternative medicine?

Viewpoint of Alternative Medicine

Alternative medicine looks at nature through a much wider lens. It is concerned with healing both the body and soul. Alternative medicine sees the beauty and power in the whole of nature and studies this in order to understand its inhabitants and their components.

The psyche is an integral part of alternative medicine. The use of this medicine also requires the spirituality of faith in which recognition and respect for both the explained and unexplained are all part of the journey of self-discovery.

Myth Four: You Can't Use It Without Proof

All ancient healing traditions possessed elements of faith. When the objectivity and detachment of scientific investigation are applied to a healing system that is based on elements of faith, the purpose of faith is missed completely. Faith does not always require a physical manifestation of its beliefs. *The purpose of faith is to believe in the unbelievable*, which is antithetical to the scientific viewpoint. This is the essence of alternative medicine that the scientific community still does not quite comprehend.

To subject alternative medicine to the same standards as conventional medicine is to ignore the scientific intractability of mind and spirit and the very intrinsic power upon which alternative medicine is founded. Empirical studies that attempt to fragment and analyze aspects of alternative medicine will never render the entire picture of how it actually works because to split it into little pieces is to alter and diminish its full power. A true understanding of alternative medicine requires simultaneous consideration of all elements of healing—the visible and invisible, the ambiguous and absolute.

Alternative medicine treatments and remedies work differently for every person and are not designed for mass application. They are also dependent on a number of variables—physical, mental, and spiritual, which, as a practical matter, are not only difficult to quantify and measure but virtually impossible to replicate at will. As such, they defy scientific control. As long as science applies its analytically detached perspective to alternative medicine, studies will yield mixed results and the true powers of alternative medicine will remain elusive.

To believe that all scientific and technological advancement is enlightened and superior and nonscientific viewpoints and provincialism are backward and inferior is absurdly naive on our part. Science cannot eliminate mystery, replace our own innate wisdom, or invalidate personal experience no matter how hard it tries. It was never intended to answer all our questions or be the sole determinant of our choices. It is not the final word on life, death, and healing.

As an object of reverence, science is a false god. It is possible, however, to respect science without worshiping it. This requires a major shift in our perception of the purpose of science and our view of health.

Science is a limited tool to help us better understand and coexist with nature on a horizontally biological level. Coexistence with nature on a vertically spiritual level can only be realized through faith. Science provides us with valuable guidelines to improve and enrich our lives. It is to life what roads are to traveling—you can get where you want to go without them but, with them, the going can be a lot smoother.

Myth Four: You Can't Use It Without Proof

We must put science into perspective, using it when appropriate but not allowing it to dominate our lives and dictate our choices. In an ideal world, a balance is struck between science and faith with both commanding equal value and respect.

Ally Versus Adversary

Science must assume a new role. It can promote peace and harmony through a better understanding of the true nature of all living systems and within a context of what is unexaminable, valuing the unexplained as it once did in its infancy. Instead of attempting to dominate and control nature by dissecting it into disconnected parts with little relationship to one another, science could consider the whole of nature in order to protect and preserve its interdependent and indivisible parts. The superficiality of a secular-based society would give way to the intimacy of a more spiritual-based one, a transition that is just beginning.

A new approach to scientific thought would allow for and honor the ambiguity and uniqueness of the human experience and all life. It would seek to illuminate the circularity of all living systems—what helps nature helps us, and what harms nature harms us. A synthesis of science and faith could delve into new arenas, elucidating the mysteries of consciousness and exploring states of awareness other than the waking, sleeping, and dreaming states we know.

6 MYTHS ABOUT ALTERNATIVE MEDICINE

To achieve these goals, new methods of research, which place greater emphasis on the value of individual experience, would be devised. Outcome studies and qualitative research, existing forms of research with this emphasis, could also be utilized.

These goals demand respect for the equality of all living things and eliminate the arrogance of our misperceived superiority over nature. A respect for nature impels us toward a reverence for all life, which is the state of being most conducive to true healing.

After all, is our effort to control nature working? Has science prevented the devastating effects of hurricanes, earthquakes, floods, fires, and plane crashes? Has it discouraged people from committing heinous acts upon each other? Has it kept children safe from harm or misfortune? Has it eliminated poverty, deprivation, and disease?

Only a few decades ago, science declared that the conquest of bacteria was forthcoming. After claims of imminent eradication, infectious disease increased almost 60% in twelve years and is now the leading cause of death worldwide. Antibiotics and other potentially harmful drugs are becoming less effective against pathogens that are constantly mutating to new and more resistant strains. Old diseases no longer respond to the old drugs, and diseases, once considered to be noninfectious, are becoming infectious. Chronic diseases, for which

Myth Four: You Can't Use It Without Proof

medical science possesses few answers, account for more than 70% of all deaths in our country.

It is indeed sobering to consider that we may have created more disease than we have cured as medically induced and environmental illness becomes more and more prevalent. With little consideration for the consequences of our actions, our planet has been irresponsibly poisoned with the beliefs that more, bigger, and faster is better, greed is good for business, and convenience always improves our lives. It is hardly enlightened to destroy the very environment that supports and sustains us and is fundamental to our very survival.

These attitudes and resulting actions diminish faith rather than enhance it. In this way, our preference for reason over faith has led us into more darkness than light.

Although technology, the offshoot of science, has provided us with many conveniences, it appears to be losing ground over its attempt to control nature. The more we try to control it through the use of technology, the less we appear to be *in* control of it. As a dynamic force undergoing constant change, nature surprises us with new and unexpected turns.

An unbridled science is not the answer nor is an obsession with all things scientific. To dismiss that which defies scientific validation as insignificant may turn out, in the long run, to be more primitive than advanced thinking.

The Power of Faith

What is dynamic and unpredictable requires faith. The natural intelligence of the body, mind, and spirit has the facility for recovery and healing and is the foundation upon which alternative medicine was created. Holistic medical systems tell us that our complex immune system is far more efficient than any medicine at combating dangerous foreign invaders.

Ironically, medical scientists have spent billions of dollars in the past discovering agents that destroy rather than improve the immune system's ability to function properly in order to treat disease. Chemotherapeutic agents are a good example of this. Realizing their error, scientists are now studying the immune system's healing potential and trying to find ways to support and enhance it. Our natural immunity is finally being recognized as one of our greatest healing resources.

The mind and spirit are also an inseparable part of our natural immunity, and we can utilize them to change our physiology through changes in our perceptions, to intuit on a deep level what we need for healing, and to maintain hope in the presence of adversity. We can change our perceptions by realizing that we choose them in the first place.

Many experts speculate that the power of the mind and spirit are responsible for 50% or more of the healing process. Using the psyche to effect

Myth Four: You Can't Use It Without Proof

change in our health involves the powers of suggestion, intuition, and faith, but cultivating these natural qualities is not easy in an environment that seeks to diminish or negate them.

The power of suggestion presents a unique opportunity in the healing process. In medical science, the power of suggestion is represented by the placebo effect, which is based on the premise that the mind affects the body. The placebo effect is defined as the beneficial results, physiological or psychological, from the use of inert medications. For example, a person takes a pill to ease pain unaware that it is only made of sugar.

Research has shown that when a toxic medicine is administered with a harmless agent and the toxic medicine is removed, the body continues to respond as though the medicine were still present. Although science is based on the elimination of the placebo effect, alternative medicine recognizes it as a great power.

Intuition or instinct is also an integral part of the healing process, but it has traditionally been viewed by science as an element of weakness or an object of contempt. "You're thinking with your heart, not your head;" "You're imagining things;" and "It's just a coincidence." These are just a few of the disparaging and dismissive ways that this natural ability is regarded by medical doctors.

Science is also responsible for objectifying and compartmentalizing intuition by associating it with only one side of the brain and by giving us the impression it has little or no value in our lives. We can use intuition, however, to determine what we need and do not need for healing, which provides us with the confidence to follow our convictions and take appropriate action to implement change.

Faith in a treatment, oneself, others, or a higher power is an important determinant of health, probably more so than any external intervention. The most common faith is faith in a higher power. It is estimated that 95% of the population believes in a higher power. Research on belief and prayer has shown that hope is a healing agent, but feeling victimized in the face of adversity and challenge is not.

Faith is emerging as an important healing tool, and more and more studies are being conducted on the healing power of belief and prayer. Some experts suggest that 90% of illness could be resolved by faith alone. If the majority of illness could be eliminated by faith, shouldn't it warrant our serious attention?

Whether it involves the power of suggestion, implemented by alternative techniques such as guided imagery; the power to intuit, cultivated by alternative practices such as meditation and breathwork; or the power of faith, exemplified by our spiritual beliefs and practice, our own untapped wisdom is inestimable in its ability to facilitate

Myth Four: You Can't Use It Without Proof

change. A critical component of every ancient wisdom tradition, faith when activated or realized can unlock many doors to healing that we never thought possible.

When we are able to recognize and develop these natural abilities through a recognition of our physical, mental, and spiritual potential, individual experience will be valued and the need for scientific proof on every subject will dissipate. The more we trust our inherent selves, the less dependent we will be on the results of scientific studies.

Be Smart

Do not cast aside an alternative medicine intervention for the sole reason that it lacks the stamp of scientific approval. You do not need the approval of science in order to benefit from an alternative intervention, as long as you choose wisely and stick with practices that have been around a long time and practitioners who know what they are doing. It will take decades for science to get there if it does at all. Although it can be an arduous process, informed and responsibly conducted trial and error is a valid approach to using this medicine.

In conventional medicine, treatments that are the objects of studies are usually new and untried, and drugs are made from highly converted materials and synthetic sources. After the effectiveness of the treatment or drug has been established, it takes even longer to get the necessary approvals to release it to the public through a medical doctor's prescription.

Alternative medicine is not new. The established practices have existed for hundreds or even thousands of years. No medicine could possibly last this long if it was ineffective or inherently harmful. The alternative treatments, remedies, herbs, and supplements that are the objects of studies are already available to the public through practitioners and the retailers who sell them.

When you use alternative medicine, do not confuse your instinct with your emotion. To avoid this common problem takes awareness and practice. In the face of serious illness, emotions frequently cloud not only your judgment but also your innate sense of what to do. Do not make health decisions out of a desperate need to stay alive. Make them out of an empowered desire to further the cause of true healing.

Be willing to be your own guide on the use of alternative medicine, trusting your instinct with equal respect for your intellect. We were given the powers of intellect and faith with the intention that we benefit from utilizing both these resources. To ignore one over the other is simply like trying to walk with only one leg. After a while, the unused leg will atrophy to the point at which we do not remember having used it at all. Albert Einstein said, "We should take care not to make the intellect

Myth Four: You Can't Use It Without Proof

our god; it has, of course, powerful muscles but no personality."

Guidelines for the Use of Unproven Alternative Therapies

1. Keep in mind that an alternative medicine practice, technique, or remedy may be effective even if it has not been proven so by scientific study.

2. Use only those alternative practices that are established such as acupuncture, homeopathy, massage, etc.

3. Remember that informed trial and error is a valid method for using alternative medicine.

4. Develop *personal health care power*, which will help you to make informed and responsible health care choices. (See Myth 1.)

5. Use common sense and sound judgment when navigating the alternative medicine waters. (See Myth 2.)

6. Do not be ruled by your emotions when making health care decisions.

6 MYTHS ABOUT ALTERNATIVE MEDICINE

People have grown weary of the powerlessness imposed upon them by the limiting belief of science, which claims that all answers to healing exist outside of ourselves. We no longer want to be shackled by its whims. Science does not answer all our questions, but faith does. Science can only be regarded as a positive endeavor to the extent that it does not cause us to mistrust or lose faith in ourselves.

When health professionals allege that we cannot use alternative medicine without scientific validation, they imply that we do not have the ability to determine for ourselves what makes us feel better or what is in our best interests. This disempowering admonition crushes the faith that we need to heal instead of enriching it. If something like this is said to you, get a second opinion—*your own*!

People want to put faith back into the process of healing. Someday we will realize that physical disease is merely a manifestation and reflection of our hearts and minds, our spiritual and mental natures. Our body is a canvas upon which our souls are written, and illness is the result rather than the cause of what ails us.

Instead of being defined as separate, distinguishable parts of a whole, health will someday be defined as the whole of inseparable parts. Without the need for qualifying monikers like "alternative," "conventional," or "integrated," all health

Myth Four: You Can't Use It Without Proof

care will automatically include simultaneous consideration for these important aspects of health
and will be called simply medicine.

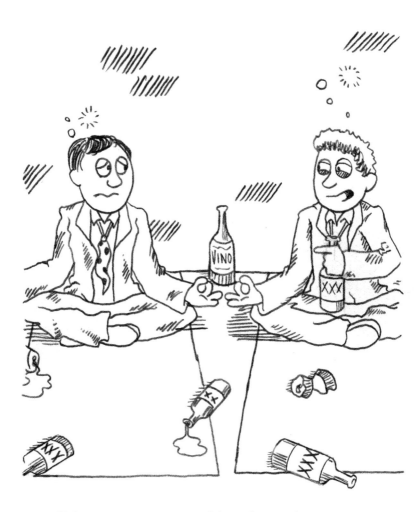

"My yoga practice is . . . *hic* . . . better than yours!"

MYTH 5

It's a Good Substitute
for Conventional Medicine

*Compromise makes a good umbrella
but a poor roof.*

JAMES RUSSELL LOWELL

Alternative medicine is primarily based on the indigenous healing practices of Eastern cultures whose view of health is very different from our own. There is a good reason why writer Rudyard Kipling wrote, "East is East and West is West, and never the twain shall meet."

The belief that alternative medicine is a good substitute for conventional medicine is a complicated one and perhaps the most controversial of all the misconceptions. The basis for this belief is that there is no adverse outcome from applying a medicine from one culture to another with differing views on health and the purpose of medicine.

This myth may be confusing to the person who wants to use alternative medicine. After all, isn't it better to substitute a more benign, natural treatment for an invasive and potentially harmful one?—only if the medicine is used the way it was intended to be used.

When we substitute alternative medicine for conventional medicine, we are using it within the context of our conventional view of health. The Western view of physical cure, however, is very different from the Eastern view of healing.

Western View of Physical Cure

With a tendency to look to external sources to meet internal needs, conventional medicine is used with the expectation that the medicine (or the one who dispenses it) is the source of healing. Medicine provides the answers and solves our problems. As a result of this view, an overdependence on medicine and intervention is created rather than a reliance on our own innate abilities, placing more faith in medicine than ourselves and more focus on cure than true healing. This leads to the objectification of the health care consumer, who plays a minor role in this process.

The objectification of the consumer breeds detachment by all parties concerned in the health

Myth Five: *It's a Good Substitute for Conventional Medicine*

care system. Spirit, mind, and disease are regarded as separate from the body, which also consists of separate, treatable parts. Detachment makes us feel more victimized than empowered by illness, which causes us to focus more on intervention than prevention and to value the treatment of illness over the maintenance of health. The Western approach to health makes it is easy for us to regard illness as an event that is outside of our control and to relinquish that control to others.

Detachment in the health care process also creates a dependence on seeking the immediate relief of symptoms rather than long-term resolution of health imbalances, which requires more extensive examination into their underlying causes. Our intolerance for inconvenience and incapacitation and our desire to avoid self-introspection at all costs makes this possible.

In the Western view, it is easier to take a pill to alleviate symptoms of illness after they arise than to develop and practice regular preventive measures before illness occurs. Taking a pill is also easier than taking a good look in the mirror. The casualties of temporary, feel-good cures are not only our health but insight, awareness, growth, and wisdom.

An overdependence on medicine leads to the excessive use of medicine, further inhibiting our full participation in the healing process. It is common knowledge that drugs and surgery are employed by doctors far more than is really necessary. The excessive use of medicine also generates consumer buying frenzies such as those that accompanied the introduction of the drugs Prozac for depression and Viagra for sexual impotence.

With a strong societal emphasis on athletic prowess and image, medicine is frequently used for purposes other than to seek relief from illness. Athletes use steroids to improve their sports performance, and women get silicone breast implants to augment their physical appearance.

There is little tolerance for ambiguity in the Western view of physical cure. There is an emotional need to label and pathologize people in order to treat them, sometimes to the point at which they become their disease and are only known in this context. People have either a diagnosable condition or no diagnosable condition; there is no in between in the conventional medical system.

Symptoms in the absence of a diagnosable illness do not exist in the Western medical lexicon, in the same way that a treatment that fails to produce the same result for the majority of people within the confines of a clinical trial is deemed ineffective by science. This can and often does result in misdiagnosis.

Eastern View of Healing

In the Eastern view of healing, *you* are the source of healing, not the medicine or another person.

Myth Five: It's a Good Substitute for Conventional Medicine

Doctors and medicine only serve to facilitate and encourage an inherent healing process you already possess.

Health is within your control and does not exist outside of you because body, mind, and spirit are inseparable and are treated accordingly. You are empowered rather than victimized by illness and the healing process because of the remarkable opportunity for growth and change that they present.

In this view, the emphasis is on the maintenance of health rather than the treatment of illness, and you play the major role in this process, not a secondary one. A healthy interdependence on healers and medicine is created. Since more faith is placed on you than on external intervention and more value is ascribed to your feelings, beliefs, and opinions, health care relationships of depth and intimacy are developed. This is the opposite of the objectification and detachment that dominates the Western approach to health.

Ambiguity is accepted as a normal part of health, and conditions are characterized in less rigid terms such as "imbalance." Instead of temporary, feel-good cures, lasting results are sought through a willingness to investigate the underlying causes of illness, no matter how painful or difficult they may be.

This goal necessitates extensive evaluation and treatment because the Eastern approach assumes that there are not just one but numerous layers of an imbalance to uncover and resolve. Multiple

6 Myths About Alternative Medicine

layers of an imbalance can also warrant multiple interventions at different stages of the healing process. There is no one "miracle cure."

Since the goal is permanent resolution, alternative medicine is designed to work on a much deeper level than conventional medicine. Symptoms may be alleviated quickly, but more often than not, they take a long time to resolve completely. One symptom may give way to another symptom, and symptoms can become much worse before they improve. The Eastern view is that if you focus solely on the alleviation of symptoms, they will become temporarily repressed only to inevitably resurface somewhere else in the body in a manner that is increasingly difficult to resolve.

Great care is taken to select the right treatment or remedy for your individual needs, eliminating the generic prescription of medicine for mass consumption and the risk of its excessive or improper use. Sometimes, an intervention in alternative medicine is no intervention at all. Doing nothing in order to allow a previous intervention to work, to give the body a chance to rest, or to encourage the body's natural inclination to right itself on its own is a powerful intervention in and of itself. Hippocrates confirmed the value of this tactic when he wrote, "To do nothing is also a good remedy."

Investigating the underlying causes of illness, uncovering and resolving the numerous layers of healing, and giving alternative medicine

Myth Five: It's a Good Substitute for Conventional Medicine

the opportunity to work properly takes time. No matter what anyone tells you, there is no quick fix to this process.

Is It Still Alternative Medicine?

Alternative medicine is very different in its approach, attitudes, and expectations from conventional medicine, which is why it is called "alternative." This poses some interesting questions.

What happens to alternative medicine when it is applied with a conventional approach to health? Is the Western doctor or practitioner who is educated and experienced in the conventional medical viewpoint able to utilize alternative medicine to its maximum potential? Does a conventionalized alternative medicine represent a new paradigm or just the old paradigm with new tricks?

Alternative medicine is being used more and more as a substitute for conventional medicine. An alternative remedy or herb is substituted for a conventional drug. An acupuncture visit is substituted for a visit to a conventional medical doctor.

It is certainly possible to use an alternative treatment or remedy in place of a conventional treatment or drug to effect a less harmful result, and like conventional medicine, it can sometimes cause an immediate improvement in symptoms. Alternative medicine, however, is much more complicated than that.

If the goal is to alleviate superficial symptoms of illness as quickly as possible with a safer, less invasive medicine, alternative medicine will ultimately disappoint. Substituting alternative medicine for conventional medicine does not improve outcome and can limit the medicine's ability to work properly to further the healing process.

If conventional medicine is so inadequate to begin with that we would seek to replace it with something else, why do this? It is by no means a major leap forward if we use alternative medicine in this manner. *Alternative medicine used exclusively with a Western perspective toward health and cure is just another form of conventional medicine.*

Alternative medicine has already assumed many of the characteristics of conventional medicine. Alternative practices become institutionalized as they are incorporated into our health care system. They also become commercialized with their widespread popularity and resulting emphasis on profit. As alternative medicine undergoes these profound changes, its priorities become more and more confused. The lines that previously distinguished conventional medicine from alternative medicine are increasingly blurred.

Institutionalized & Commercialized Medicine

Institutionalized medicine is based on a gatekeeper mentality in which medical choices are at the

Myth Five: It's a Good Substitute for Conventional Medicine

discretion of physicians, insurance regulators, and pharmaceutical companies rather than consumers. It includes government-regulated training programs, third party involvement, and capitalized care, which involves paying a fixed, per person amount for a set of services over a specified period of time, and is exemplified by the managed competition between regulators and providers.

The institutionalization of alternative medicine is a slow but almost certain reality. More and more alternative practices are licensed, added to health insurance policies, and organized into professional associations, which subjects them to the scrutiny and control of others.

Institutionalized care applies the same medicine to anyone who fits into a specific category of medical history and symptomatology. Successful individual experiences are transformed into scientifically proven, standardized treatments and techniques, which are then applied to a mass audience. This results in the accepted practice of assembly line medicine, treating people the same regardless of their individual needs or differences.

Commercialism is defined as an "excessive emphasis on profit." It advances consumerism, which is based on the theory that an increase in the consumption of goods is economically desirable. Commercialization occurs when huge opportunities for profit exist in what is popular with a mass audience.

6 MYTHS ABOUT ALTERNATIVE MEDICINE

Whenever anything becomes popular, however, its integrity is frequently threatened or sacrificed for the sake of what will sell. This is the price we pay for living in an economically driven society. The popularity of alternative medicine increases the chance for its widespread use and acceptance, but it also increases the chance for its misinterpretation and misuse.

As a $40 billion a year industry, commercialized alternative medicine is already a reality. Its practices and products are becoming increasingly commodified. Along with advertisements for pharmaceutical drugs and laser eye surgery, there are now advertisements for various herbal remedies and homeopathy. The people who practice alternative medicine are organizing into legal corporations and business partnerships, whose priority is the financial bottom line. Alternative medicine products, nutritional supplements, and health food stores, once family-owned enterprises, have been absorbed by large conglomerates.

Growth, at least the personal kind, is not an inevitable outcome of commercialization. Complacency is, which becomes dangerous when applied to health care. "If I get an acupuncture treatment, I don't have to watch what I eat" or "I have a meditation cushion and go to retreats; therefore, I am spiritually enlightened."

A health care system based on profit is held in higher regard than the welfare of the people it serves and causes the frequent misuse of medicine. It creates

Myth Five: It's a Good Substitute for Conventional Medicine

a duality in the health care relationship and compromises your care. It is prudent to question any system of health care with this priority.

Alternative medicine is acquiring the same misplaced priorities as conventional medicine. It is fast becoming an elitist medicine in which the best providers are only available to those who can afford them since most providers either refuse to accept insurance benefits or are not eligible for them. Alternative medicine has also been externalized because its power is regarded as something that exists outside of ourselves. It has also been secularized in that only its tangible qualities are valued with disregard shown for its inherent mystical ones.

Alternative medicine began as an alternative to the materialism and detachment of conventional medicine, but it is now becoming a driving force behind maintaining the status quo.

Alternative Medicine with a Conventional View

When alternative medicine is practiced with a conventional medical view, the obvious happens. Alternative providers and treatments are viewed as the source of healing, rather than facilitators, with the expectation that they can solve our problems. Providers fail to help us utilize our own inner resources to achieve more lasting results because their beliefs and opinions are regarded as more important than our own.

6 MYTHS ABOUT ALTERNATIVE MEDICINE

Alternative interventions are used to provide immediate relief of symptoms rather than address the underlying causes of illness. They are applied to a mass audience without consideration for individual needs and with diminished results. Lifestyle, emotional, spiritual, and other relevant issues are ignored or are never raised in the first place in the interview and assessment process.

Alternative providers work no more collaboratively with one another than conventional providers. The ones who become well known charge excessive fees, making their services unavailable to the average consumer. We may be encouraged to participate in treatment we do not need or treatment a provider is unqualified to administer simply because he needs the business.

Alternative medicine is frequently described as holistic. Holistic is defined as body, mind, and spirit and the intent to address these aspects of health as a single phenomenon. In alternative medicine, physical health is not the only concern. Unfortunately, there is far more talk than actual practice of a holistic approach in alternative medicine as many alternative providers continue to treat these indivisible elements quite separately. Similar to food product claims of "all natural," just because a provider claims that his practice is holistic does not make it so.

The phrase "body, mind, and spirit" is also increasingly used as a marketing ploy to sell

Myth Five: It's a Good Substitute for Conventional Medicine

everything from allergy medicine to automobiles. It has become overused to the point at which its true meaning is obscured, reinforcing the idea that these aspects of health are really separate things.

Stories of holistic practices that are not holistic abound. A "holistic" massage therapist at a well-known health spa illegally performed a spinal adjustment on a client without a medical history, permission, or warning, resulting in serious physical injury that took years to resolve. A "holistic" orthopedic doctor, running late in his schedule, caused an appointment time of thirty minutes to be reduced to five minutes for a new client. Failing to apologize or acknowledge responsibility for his lateness and after agreeing to accept a reduced fee, he then attacked the client in a subsequent letter for having no respect for him. A holistic approach includes how you are treated as much as what you are treated with.

A few years ago, a national magazine cover featured the picture of a famous alternative medicine doctor with the caption, "Can this guy make you healthy?" This attitude perpetuates the myth that we are powerless to effect change in our own health. It results in the same dependence on providers, medicine, and intervention rather than on prevention, healthy self-care, and our own healing capacity. We become no more involved in the healing process of alternative medicine than in the physical cure sought by conventional medicine.

6 MYTHS ABOUT ALTERNATIVE MEDICINE

Many alternative medicine providers encourage the continuation of these views. Frankly, *providers who apply alternative medicine with a conventional medical viewpoint and attitude are simply not practicing alternative medicine.*

In fairness, we must share the responsibility for this attitude. We continue to defer decisions to alternative providers rather than assume responsibility ourselves. We feel victimized by illness and only seek alternative treatment when we are injured or ill, so providers continue to profit from our suffering. We use alternative methods and techniques without consideration for all aspects of our health, pressuring providers to give us a pill to resolve our symptoms rather than doing the deeper work necessary for true healing. It is no easier to practice regular prevention or take a good look in the mirror at the unpleasant or painful aspects of our lives that are impacting our health than it was before.

Since we do not want to do the necessary work, we use alternative medicine excessively by taking an inappropriate dosage of a remedy or an herb or taking it on a prolonged basis. We buy remedies solely on the basis of casual recommendations and mass media reports rather than educate ourselves about them or consult with a specialist. Like the drugs Prozac and Viagra, herbs such as St. John's wort (depression), kava kava (mood), L-tryptophan (sleep), melatonin (sleep), and 5-HTP (sleep) are

Myth Five: It's a Good Substitute for Conventional Medicine

instantly sell-outs the day after a media report touts their virtues.

Fanaticism can also apply to our use of health-promoting foods. This is exemplified by our national fixation with all things soy, despite the potential negative consequences of consuming too much of it. Korean *kimichi*, a cabbage or other vegetable fermented in herbs and spices, is another health-promoting food that is gaining in popularity.

It is also possible to use alternative medicine experiences excessively. Not unlike drug addicts, there are "New Age junkies" who go from teacher to teacher and technique to technique, spending a fortune trying all the latest therapies with the hope that someone or something will eventually resolve their dilemma. But constantly looking for relief from a teacher or technique at the expense of all else is no better than looking for relief from a pill.

People who fall into this trap and who are encouraged to do so by a billion dollar New Age industry, often become addicted to the search and the emotional incapacitation that is the impetus for it. These people are missing the point of healing altogether. The point of healing is to find out what works for you, so you can undertake the internal hard work so essential to good health, using the knowledge and awareness that comes from this inner journey to more fully participate in life.

Our desire for the quick fix and our use of alternative medicine for purposes other than healing are extended to esoteric practices such as the exceedingly popular yoga. Yoga is a philosophy and lifestyle, encompassing physical fitness, nutrition, yogic breathing, meditation, personal habits, and state of mind and requiring many years of practice to achieve proficiency.

Bending to meet our Western needs, yoga has been distilled into a mere exercise for weight-loss, anti-aging, and stress-reduction purposes. Mutations of yoga practice are created to meet these goals and are frequently taught with an aggressive, competitive approach, bearing little resemblance to the original intent and effect of traditional yogic practice. Although steeped in renunciation and asceticism, yoga has also become a magnet for retail sales, generating hundreds of thousands of dollars in profits annually and making millionaires out of many of its purveyors.

Eclectic practices may satisfy our need for variety, the spice of life, but simplicity, repetition, and consistency are the condiments of health in alternative practice.

Our conventional system does not create an environment conducive to true healing, and alternative medicine is fast becoming a part of it. The consequences are obvious. If alternative medicine does not provide immediate relief, keep our interest, or live up to expectations, we become disillusioned, abandoning the medicine and declaring it no good. It is much easier to blame the medicine than to

Myth Five: It's a Good Substitute for Conventional Medicine

acknowledge our own failure to do our part in the healing process, which includes consideration of all factors that impact health and impede the medicine's ability to work properly.

Issues That Get Ignored

Preventable lifestyle and environmental issues tend to be ignored in conventional medicine, even though they are obvious impediments to health. We are aware of their impact on our health but continue to use medicine to try to compensate for them.

Mass-processed foods, contaminated water supply, sedentary lifestyles, social isolation, unabated psychological stress, unresolved pain and traumas, substance abuse, and environmental pollution are just a few of the many problems that are unique to industrialized societies and that affect our health. Like "body, mind, and spirit," there is more talk than actual practice in addressing these issues in health care. As technology continues to be an intractable part of our daily lives, it will become more and more difficult for us to avoid facing these problems.

Alternative medicine is not a substitute for an unhealthy lifestyle. Most alternative providers will tell you that most of their clients have at least one lifestyle issue that is an impediment to their health, for which they would rather take a pill than deal with it. Alternative medicine does not compensate for a destructive relationship, an unfulfilling

6 Myths About Alternative Medicine

job, low self-esteem, a lack of rest or sleep, inadequate physical exercise, poor social skills, excessive alcohol consumption, poor nutritional habits, negativity, a lack of intimacy, or a loss of faith.

A lifestyle that is healthy is not just about eating right and getting enough exercise. It also involves attitude, awareness, and behavior and includes characteristics such as honesty, generosity, kindness, grace under fire, and service to others. If you want to use alternative medicine with any degree of success, you must engage in healthy lifestyle habits and learn to effectively manage personal and societal stress.

For example, the herb St. John's Wort has been touted by many experts as a miracle cure for depression, and many people take the herb for this reason. There is nothing wrong with using an herb to alleviate a depressed mood because it may better able you to recognize and resolve the underlying cause of the depression. The herb only serves a temporary function, however, and is not a permanent solution to the problem. An herb will not resolve destructive behavioral patterns or increase intimacy in your life, which may be the actual cause of the depression. You are responsible for addressing these issues yourself.

Health conditions can often bring your attention to an unhealthy lifestyle issue by mimicking it. For example, one woman became involved in a destructive relationship with a man whose family was

Myth Five: It's a Good Substitute for Conventional Medicine

characterized as "parasitic." After a year of trying to survive this highly contentious environment, she ultimately contracted a parasite. Another woman suffered from asthma and complained that nothing, including alternative medicine, could resolve her condition. But this woman had a well-known reputation for pettiness where money was concerned. A lack of oxygen for herself, as reflected by the asthma, seemed to symbolize her lack of generosity toward others.

Issues That Get in the Way

Intention is the great motivator, and motivation determines outcome. There are intentions that motivate us to action in Western society, which can also be deterrents to health and have a negative impact on our use of alternative medicine. These intentions are so deeply woven into the fabric of our daily lives that we barely notice the extent to which they influence our thoughts and actions. As a result of this, their effect on our use of alternative medicine is never properly considered.

Since these intentions loom over every aspect of our lives, we naturally apply them to health care. They affect our use of both conventional and alternative medicine and cause us to use the latter in a materialistic and superficial manner.

Understanding why you use alternative medicine is as important as the fact that you use it. Do you use alternative medicine to take more responsibility for your health and because it is compatible with your world view, beliefs, and values, or do you use it for more materialistic or frivolous reasons?

Ironically, the very generation credited with bringing alternative medicine into the mainstream must share responsibility for encouraging its superficial use. The baby-boom generation has turned out to be far more materialistic than the parents they complained about so vociferously in the 1960s. As serial consumers desperate to reverse the aging process, they are a driving force behind using alternative medicine for all the wrong reasons.

Using alternative medicine for materialistic or superficial reasons is more about satisfying the ego than serving the soul. It encourages a casual attachment to the surface of things in order to avoid the deeper, more complex, and sometimes darker side of life. We view everything through this lens and rely repeatedly on these motivations to make us feel better. The more we use them, the more we need them. Again, their excessive use represents a futile attempt to fill the intimate void in our lives, like trying to fill that glass with the gaping hole in the bottom.

Consider the effect of the following intentions on your use of alternative medicine, which apply to providers and consumers alike:

Myth Five: It's a Good Substitute for Conventional Medicine

• *Competition*

Alternative medicine is not intended to be used as an opportunity to compete with others. The entire point of this medicine is missed if you use it while worrying about your level of accomplishment as it compares with others. If you feel superior because your practice is more advanced than others or inferior because it is less advanced than others, the purpose of alternative medicine is not served.

Competition produces adversariness, which is not conducive to the effective use of alternative medicine, personal growth, or healing. It also promotes the notion that beginners are inferior to advanced participants. This causes people who are just starting out to jump unprepared into advanced practices simply because they do not want to be known as beginners.

There are negative consequences to participating in any activity without adequate preparation. It can make you feel inferior, and you also risk subjecting yourself to serious harm. Taking on more than you are prepared to deal with is also counterproductive. For example, there are more benefits to performing a beginning yoga pose well than an advanced pose poorly.

Competition may encourage physical or intellectual accomplishment but not emotional or spiritual advancement. Save it for the playing field because competition does not belong in health care. Although it is blasphemous in a capitalistic society to suggest that competition is bad, it is reasonable to suggest that it can be misused or taken to a level that is clearly unhealthy. It can also contribute to the intentions listed below.

- *Acquisitionism*

    Acquiring alternative medicine experiences and merchandise does not improve your use of this medicine. In the New Age movement, acquisitionism is sometimes disguised as a vehicle to personal growth and happiness. Collecting books, statues, meditation aids, yoga props, workshops or retreats, gurus, and alternative treatment experiences is just another form of materialism, like collecting stamps or fine art.

    Owning New Age paraphernalia does not automatically mean that you use alternative medicine for material reasons. Only if you value yourself and others based on these acquisitions is the use of alternative medicine materially motivated.

    Using alternative medicine for solely cosmetic reasons or with unrealistic expectations

Myth Five: It's a Good Substitute for Conventional Medicine

about its ability to avert the natural aging process is just another form of materialism. You can also be spiritually materialistic. This type of acquisitionism presumes that spiritual activities are superior to material ones, but it is really only the flip side of the same coin.

Acquisitionism directed toward others is exploitive, and alternative medicine is never to be used in this manner. Using alternative medicine to gain popularity, money, notoriety, power, and control is antithetical to its purpose. This pertains to the currently popular use of spirituality for commercial purposes, such as to sell products, get higher ratings on broadcast shows, or entertain the masses.

In spiritual practice, many teachers believe there should be no required payment for services, only donations based on the student's ability to pay. They claim that if charges are imposed, the benefits of the practice will be lost altogether.

• *Popularity*

In a consumer-driven culture, there is a natural tendency for us to be attracted to the prevailing fashion, and alternative medicine now fits easily into this category. There is a distinct difference between engaging in a practice *because* it is the latest trend and engaging in it *even though* it is the latest trend.

Alternative medicine is not intended to be used to satisfy your need for social acceptance, although fellowship, a positive endeavor with demonstrated health benefits, can result from its use. Using alternative medicine because it is popular has limited value.

Avoiding superficiality and materialism in alternative medicine is about taking responsibility for your life in the absence of external gratifications. In order to increase the effectiveness of alternative medicine, you must be willing to examine your reasons for using it. Some interesting answers may arise from this line of inquiry.

Two Different Alternative Medicines

The dichotomy between the Western and Eastern points of view has resulted in two distinct groups of alternative medicine providers—those who want to keep it out of the hands of institutionalized medicine and those who do not.

One of the fears of the former is that conventional medicine is taking over alternative medicine, which will be administered by providers with little

Myth Five: It's a Good Substitute for Conventional Medicine

or no understanding of it. As a result of this, alternative medicine will become an inextricable part of the same inefficient and unresponsive bureaucratic quagmire that plagues our health care system today. Medical doctors and scientists, however, want to translate the precepts of alternative medicine into ones that they can understand within the context of conventional medical training and to which they can apply the Western paradigm of health.

A consequence of the latter is "crash course" alternative medicine with medical doctors and scientists attempting to reduce this medicine into neat, definable packages that can be easily learned. Another consequence is that a predominating medical science will continue to dictate our alternative medicine choices rather than empower us to make our own choices, which is so integral to the use of this medicine.

The result of these two viewpoints is the existence of two different alternative medicines—the one practiced by conventional doctors who are trained in the Western view of physical cure and the one practiced by alternative medicine purists who are trained in the Eastern view of healing. The choice is yours.

A Different Approach

We may be able to do little to change the economic priority in health care, but we can use alternative

6 Myths About Alternative Medicine

medicine with a different attitude and expectation from the ones we use for conventional medicine.

An expanded view of health is the environment most conducive to healing. In this view, health is only a state of mind, so illness does not always include physical incapacity. Illness is also a normal part of life and can cause us to change for the better. Our bodies have the capacity to heal on their own without any intervention, and in most cases, this is what will happen. But, sometimes, this natural ability is impeded, and interventions must be employed to encourage it.

When our healing capacity is compromised and the compromise results in illness, regaining a state of health can be a long and complex process. Illness is often wisdom struggling for our attention and a symptom of a much larger issue. We can regard illness as an impediment or an extraordinary opportunity for learning and growth. We can feel alienated and victimized by illness or blessed by it. We can feel inadequate or empowered by the struggle to be well.

Perception is a choice, and we can choose to perceive illness positively or negatively. Alternative medicine will never live up to its potential until we change the way we view health. Changing our view of health will change our view of everything.

Our goal should be healing, not merely cure, and we need to be willing to go anywhere we need to go to experience it because there is little room for

Myth Five: It's a Good Substitute for Conventional Medicine

denial in the effective use of alternative medicine. It does not involve giving power away to another person, medical intervention, or treatment. It does require a thorough investigation and evaluation of the deeper, often hidden causes of illness, a process which takes both time and effort. Allowing alternative medicine to work properly also takes time and effort. It will facilitate lasting results only if it is used with a commitment to true healing.

Guidelines for the Effective Use of Alternative Medicine

The primary methods for getting the most out of alternative medicine and using it the way it was intended to be used include the following:

1. Take an active role in the health care relationship.

2. Be discriminating about the alternative practices and providers that you use by selecting practices appropriate for your circumstances and providers who practice for the right reasons.

3. Use alternative interventions responsibly with the understanding that different ones may be required for different levels or stages of healing, no intervention may be the best

6 MYTHS ABOUT ALTERNATIVE MEDICINE

> course of action, and symptoms may get worse before getting better.
>
> 4. Be willing to address all aspects of health, especially those issues that you most want to avoid or that are the most painful to you.
>
> 5. Develop healthy lifestyle habits and reasons for using alternative medicine other than to compete with others, to acquire things, experiential or material, or to be fashionable.

Just as our compulsion toward hero worship may be more about filling the void created by an absence of intimacy than a genuine search for answers, the billions of dollars spent each year on alternative medicine may be more about a continuation of our search for the quick fix than a newly evolved self-reliance. The great irony of the Western world is that while grasping for the latest technological development, we are simultaneously grasping for the latest herbal remedy to fill the void that our very dependence on technology creates. The Westernization of alternative medicine is a reflection of our health care system, which is merely a reflection of ourselves.

When we expand our knowledge and awareness to embrace a larger picture of health, we will learn

Myth Five: It's a Good Substitute for Conventional Medicine

to use alternative medicine as a powerful new ally to advance our own natural ability to heal rather than as a replacement for something else. Alternative medicine is different from conventional medicine. If we continue to use alternative medicine as a substitute for conventional medicine, it will become just another form of conventional medicine, losing its intrinsic value and benefits.

When we assume a larger role and take more responsibility for our health, we also create a new paradigm of health and approach to healing. To experience true healing is the intention best served in order to optimize the effectiveness and preserve the intrinsic value of alternative medicine. When we use alternative medicine for the right reasons and these important qualities remain intact, the benefits of using this medicine are clearly maximized.

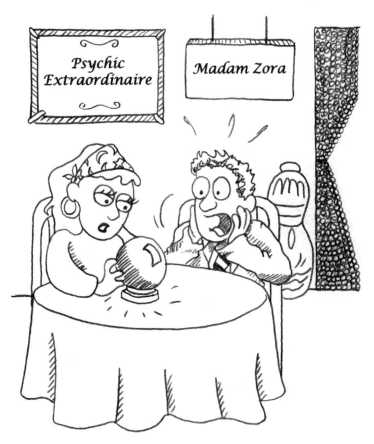

"In your next life, you will be married to your mother-in-law."   "Oh no!!!"

MYTH 6

Spirit is Always Positive

If you believe, no proof is necessary. If you don't believe, no proof is sufficient.

The holistic nature of alternative medicine involves a natural focus on spirit and the search for deeper meaning. This aspect of healing cannot be separated or removed from its use. New Age idealism and the commercialization of spirituality often lead to the mistaken belief that spirit is only positive and represents everything that is warm and fuzzy in the universe. Although it is certainly about angels and light, spirit can also be about demons and darkness.

The negative in spirit refers to complex issues, about which very little is known. As a result, the negative in spirit does not receive the attention it deserves in the health care process, and its impact on our health goes unrecognized.

Spirit is the essence of our being and keeper of our soul. It would be impossible to have any discussion about healing without consideration for its spiritual meaning. If there is a power in the universe greater than the one we know, common sense dictates that there are spiritual aspects of healing that may also be beyond our immediate awareness. After all, good people with healthy lifestyles, attitudes, and environments get sick too.

Let us look at it from a purely intellectual standpoint. We accept that there exists positive and negative in the physical: the positive is represented by physical fitness, and the negative is represented by physical illness or injury. We accept that there exists positive and negative in the mental: the positive is represented by kindness and compassion, and the negative is represented by the shadow side of personality. In a truly holistic approach to health, the existence of positive and negative in the physical and mental also points to the existence of positive and negative in the spiritual.

New Attention to Spirit

There may be little understanding of spirituality because its ethereal nature defies scientific study and explanation with any degree of certainty,

Myth Six: Spirit is Always Positive

clarity, or specificity. As a billion dollar-a-year industry, there is certainly renewed interest in it.

Books on spirituality top the national bestseller lists. Although book sales in general have increased only 3% in the past few years, those on spirituality have increased an estimated 20%. There are also constant references to spirituality in the media and numerous news programs, television shows, and movies on spirituality, the paranormal, and the supernatural.

There is both a good and bad side to this renewed interest. Many people want to become reconnected to their spirituality in a genuine desire to lead more authentic lives. As a result of its popularity, however, spirituality is exploited more than any other aspect of alternative medicine, and because there is some work involved in realizing spirituality, we talk about it more than we live it.

Spiritual practices are founded on the principles of poverty, sacrifice, and renunciation. But spirituality has become a hot commodity on the retail market, thanks to our insatiable consumerism and despite the fact that it cannot be bought or sold. As the catchword for everything wonderful, the word spirit is used and overused to the point at which its true meaning is trivialized and diminished, turning it into something it is not.

Although an integral part of alternative medicine and the frequent topic of discussion, spirit and its effect on the body and mind are rarely mentioned in the health interview. One thing is certain—treating spiritual impediments to health requires exceptional knowledge and skill.

Spirit Defined

Spirit *is* the big picture. It refers to an expanded or heightened awareness and symbolizes the connectedness of life and its larger meaning and purpose. It is about your relationship with the divine and all things mystical and mysterious. Spirit is the discovery of your true or essential nature and the search for inner peace, balance, and harmony. As such, it is an intensely personal experience.

True spirituality is never used for self-aggrandizement, only for enlightenment. It can be neither acquired like a possession nor easily explained. Spiritual openings occur on a physical, mental, or spiritual level and often in the presence of adversity and suffering. Spirituality exists in the face of strength and vulnerability and is realized through the development of an inner life, which is achieved through hard work and daily practice.

Although we think spirit exists only in positive experiences, there is spirit in every experience, good and bad. We tacitly accept the role of fate when something fortunate happens to us, often describing it as "lucky" or "destined." But when something bad happens, we desperately ask, "Why is this happening to

Myth Six: Spirit is Always Positive

me?" or "What went wrong?" and approach the situation with fear, bitterness, or anger.

It is easy to credit the cosmos when things are going well but not as easy when things are going wrong. This is the time, however, when recognizing the bigger picture matters the most and provides the greatest opportunity for growth and change. When you are connected to spirit, your experiences may not be different but your view of them is.

Spirituality is not synonymous with religion. Spirit is innate and fluid, and religion is a creation of man and, as such, can be very static. Religion is typically man's interpretation of faith and the word and life of a prophet or group. It is represented by theory, hierarchy, and dogma and is frequently taught through metaphor, legend, and exaggeration. As such, religion may not reflect the prophet's original intentions. For example, many Biblical experts now believe that Mary Magdalen was a revered disciple of Christ, not a prostitute, a characterization promulgated by Pope Gregory in the sixth century to exclude women from leadership roles in the patriarchal Catholic Church.

When usurped by ideological and fanatical elements, religion becomes a distortion of spirituality, driven by fear, greed, control, shame, judgment, and guilt rather than love. Zealots often use religion as justification to injure or kill others, the antithesis of spirituality.

6 MYTHS ABOUT ALTERNATIVE MEDICINE

Although religion frequently personifies hypocrisy, spirit always represents truth. It is possible to be religious but not spiritual, spiritual but not religious, and both religious and spiritual.

Spiritual Materialism

Spirit is characterized by a deeper awareness and an understanding of our true nature, essence, or soul's purpose, but it often gets translated into a particular philosophy, which can then be read, studied, performed, heard, or taught. With a societal focus on the individual over the common good, spirit can also become relegated to the confines of individual accomplishment. An epidemic of self-importance in our society and the potential for commercial exploitation feed this focus.

The acquisition of spirit in the form of material and experiential excess is believed, promoted, and sold. This is not spirituality; it is *spiritual materialism*.

Our society encourages the translation of spirit into mediocre and superficial terms. We try to analyze it because we think there is an explanation for everything. But language is a device of mankind and is subject to its rules and regulations. As such, words can never capture the true nature of creativity and the divine.

We also become attached to religious doctrine along with its rules and rituals, forgetting that they are only the means to an end and not the end itself.

Myth Six: *Spirit is Always Positive*

Devotion to a spiritual practice or knowledge of its dogma does not necessarily result in consciousness in thought and deed or spiritual awareness. On the other hand, the lack of it does not always point to spiritual ignorance or depravity.

Spirit in theory is different from spirit in practice. Spirit in practice is about whom a person is, not what he says or does. Spiritual materialism is derived from the latter, but spiritual knowledge can only emerge and be cultivated from silence and solitude. Ancient wisdom traditions characterize spirituality as something that "cannot be known but can only be."

An emphasis on saying or doing reduces the most profound experience to casual anecdote. Writer Ernest Hemingway recounted a story about World War II soldiers who felt emotionally diminished after telling others about their war experiences. Doing is helpful to a certain point, especially in the form of service toward others, but it will not ultimately get you where you need to go for true healing.

There can be no doubt that the commodification of spirituality is profane. Although purveyors of New Age products and services would have you believe otherwise, you do not need special accouterments, props, or languages to realize spirituality because it lies within you. When you come to know it, a sense of spirituality in daily life is automatically cultivated and the divinity in all living things is recognized.

6 Myths About Alternative Medicine

There is no need to worry about your level of spiritual accomplishment or to dwell on what others are doing or what they know. It is far more important to live authentically with a loving heart and to apply it to your daily life than to talk about or engage in spiritual practice for superficial reasons. This is *applied spirituality*.

If the intention behind engaging in spiritual practice is for material or superficial reasons, its benefits will be diminished or lost altogether. Using spirituality for superficial purposes is the equivalent of continuing to seek and grasp for worldly gratifications. Seekers of true healing use spiritual practice with a broader view and a willingness to find their own voice rather than imitate the voices of others.

Spirit & Illness

Spirit is difficult to conceptualize as it relates to health. The Western view is that the primary cause of illness is physical, which is based on the belief that we have power over nature, and disease is an enemy that can be eradicated.

Ancient healing traditions believe that the primary cause of illness is spiritual, which is based on the premise that physical health comprises only a fraction of the picture and illness provides opportunities for learning and growth. Although these ancient traditions did not arise from technologically

Myth Six: Spirit is Always Positive

advanced societies, it is a mistake to assume that they are inferior to us in other ways.

A spiritual basis for illness holds that although illness may present itself in the physical body, something else warrants our attention. Illness is merely a manifestation of a deeper, underlying cause. In this view, fate is given great value and there are no accidents in life. People who survive an unexplainable, tragic event understand this concept implicitly.

Fate is not the equivalent of victimization or loss of free will and does not involve the ego. Fate has to do with the inevitable forces of nature and the lessons to be learned from surrendering to those forces. To surrender to the divine forces of nature is to have loving trust toward an experience and a more meaningful view of life.

In the face of adversity, it is pointless to ask, "What could I have done to avoid this experience?" This attitude only produces regret, and regret, a function of ego, does not promote healing. Ego is like a closed venetian blind that blocks out the sunlight with not only regret but fear, judgment, guilt, anger, and even sorrow. When ego is involved, there is always something to protect, which distracts from the meaning of an experience. Regret also presumes that there is no value in an experience and all matters are within your immediate control, giving no credit to a higher power.

6 MYTHS ABOUT ALTERNATIVE MEDICINE

In the face of adversity, it is more beneficial to ask, "What did I learn from this experience?" and to acknowledge that you are part of the larger picture.

A belief in the separateness of things is illusory and also a function of ego. Everything that exists is connected to everything else. This connectedness is often referred to as subtle energy, which is generated by all living matter.

Evidence of our spiritual connectedness exists all around us. Have you ever thought about someone who suddenly called, sensed a person in a room before seeing him, or knew what someone would say before he said it? Did you concidentally receive a book that spoke to an unresolved problem or a message that encouraged helpful reflection? What about the times you sensed something was not right or were thwarted in a way that ultimately turned out to be to your benefit?

Everyone remembers having a serendipitous experience, especially if it is a positive one. If we were aware of the fundamental part spirit plays in everyday life, there would be no question as to the part it plays in illness.

The Physical World

Spiritual healing manifests itself in many ways. At its core, it involves being in the presence of love in all its forms. Being in the presence of love is being

Myth Six: Spirit is Always Positive

uplifted through culturally artistic pleasure, the beauty of nature, the miracle of birth, and inspiring people who embody qualities such as kindness and compassion.

Spiritual healing triggers increased awareness and change that would not occur if you remained physically well. You may experience a change in your perception, behavior, relationships, or physical environment; learn to utilize inner resources as guidance for what is helpful and harmful for healing; renew lost connections with nature, animals, and people; or acquire faith in a higher power.

Spiritual healing is encouraged by awakening to the unseen parts of your life, termed the shadow side of personality. It is also realized by slowing down, simplifying your life, surrounding yourself with silence, giving attention to the breath, listening to yourself through prayer, learning the nature of the mind through meditation, and helping others. Learning to be fully in the present moment and to extend kindness and forgiveness to others, especially in difficult times, are important components of spiritual health.

There is joy in these experiences, but there can also be pain and sorrow in the very same experiences. What is one person's pleasure is another's pain. Although there is value in having spiritually pleasurable experiences, the potential for learning and growth is severely limited in the presence of pleasure alone. This is the reason spiritual healing frequently occurs in the face of catastrophic experiences such as serious illness.

There is no pleasure without pain, no good without bad, no love without hate, and no light without dark. Darkness is just another form of light in which moments of increased awareness, wisdom, and healing are possible.

The Spirit World

Spiritual healing involves more than merely finding joy in sorrow or finding happiness in the presence of difficult circumstances. Spiritual healing can also be about more complex life lessons and tasks. To understand this, it is important to be able to distinguish between spiritual issues from the perspective of the physical world and spiritual issues from the perspective of the spirit world.

Spiritual issues from the perspective of the physical world involve conditions within our immediate awareness. Spiritual issues from the perspective of the spirit world involve conditions outside of our immediate awareness and are difficult to understand from a physical world perspective. Spirit world issues are often mistakenly perceived as being exclusively benevolent because their resolution is so complex and few people possess the skill to resolve them.

Common sense dictates that if there are physical and mental aspects of spirituality, there are also

Myth Six: Spirit is Always Positive

spiritual aspects of spirituality. It would then follow that if there are both positive and negative aspects of spirituality in the physical world, there are also positive and negative aspects of spirituality in the spirit world.

Spiritual issues from the perspective of the spirit world are usually described as metaphysical, paranormal, or supernatural. They are termed psi and include events such as telepathy, visions, precognitive dreams, out-of-body experiences, visitations by angels or spirits, conversations with God, and experiences with radiant or divine light.

Spirit world issues sometimes involve a spiritual opening or vulnerability to an imbalance, which is connected to negative energetic forces such as those represented by the seven deadly sins of pride, avarice, lust, anger, gluttony, envy, and sloth. They can relate to the loss of part or all of the soul, karmic consequences or deeds from a past lifetime, a damaged psyche, a shamanic curse, ancestral contracts and programs, sacred contracts made before birth, the wrath of nature, and even spiritual possession. (One Brazilian spiritual healer claims the latter comprises 80–90% of his work.) In the extreme, spirit world issues can be about the presence of disembodied spirits or ghosts, occult energies, extraterrestrials, and other entities.

Spirit world issues occur for a variety of reasons and are associated with a person's thoughts, attitudes, and behavior. Action and thought produce energy according to the spirit world perspective and having an open mind about spiritual phenomena automatically makes you more vulnerable to their effects.

Strong emotion such as fear or trauma creates a vulnerability to a spiritual imbalance. A weakened physical, emotional, or spiritual condition caused by illness, a longing, alcohol or drug use, marital disruption, past actions, and a sudden loss of faith also creates an opening to an imbalance. Spending time in hospitals, funeral homes, and cemeteries exposes a person to possible spiritual imbalance.

A spiritual imbalance can result in a physical or mental imbalance and subsequent illness. There are many well-educated, intelligent people who believe that spiritual imbalance is a common occurrence in the human condition.

Spiritual Resolution

Just as there are individual differences in physical and emotional immunity, there are also individual differences in spiritual immunity. Some people possess the ability to resist or avoid a spiritual imbalance better than others. Like physical and emotional immunity, this resistance is also based on a variety of factors such as your level of awareness, a willingness to learn life lessons, the ability to protect yourself, and the strength of your faith.

Myth Six: Spirit is Always Positive

Not only can a spiritual imbalance result in physical illness, but physical illness can also bring about a spiritual imbalance. Thoughts and actions make you vulnerable to spiritual imbalance, but spiritual imbalance can also influence your thoughts and actions.

Symptoms of a spiritual imbalance can also be very subtle. A persistence of disturbing thoughts or feelings that are without explanation or provocation may signal a spiritual imbalance. Recurring, unexplainable nightmares, involuntary behavior, or an unusual number of unexplainable adversities may also point to a spiritual imbalance.

Resolution of a spiritual imbalance is complicated and usually requires a practitioner of extraordinary talents. Earthly interventions include the use of herbs, crystals, ritual offerings, smudging, prayer, meditation, trance, chanting, pilgrimage, behavior modification, hypnosis, psychotherapy, and alternative treatments like acupuncture. Many spiritual healing traditions also rely on the healing power of angels, ancestral spirits, spirit helpers, and spirit guides, in addition to earthly intervention, to restore an individual to a state of balance.

Spirit world interventions are often employed in a formal ritual or ceremony. Spiritual healers sometimes journey to the spirit world by entering into an altered state in order to effect change in the physical world and the condition of the person seeking help.

6 MYTHS ABOUT ALTERNATIVE MEDICINE

You can build your spiritual immunity and resist an imbalance by strengthening the energy field that surrounds you, commonly known as your aura. The primary ways to do this are:

- Control negative thoughts and actions. Do psychological work to remedy negative patterns of thought and behavior, excessive and persistent states of mind, or any mental condition that depletes your energy field.

- Avoid excessive alcohol or drug use, which depletes your energy field and makes you vulnerable to a psychic attack. Avoid the consumption of pork, which is also believed to lower your vibrational level.

- Balance your energy centers or *chakras* with treatments such as external *qigong* and crystal baths, which cleanse your energy field.

- Engage in regular contemplative practice, such as prayer or meditation, to connect to what is termed higher or god-consciousness to strengthen your energy field.

- Avoid situations in the physical environment that have an adverse impact on your energy field, such as the use of electric blankets and living in close proximity to power lines or plants.

Myth Six: Spirit is Always Positive

- Utilize props that have a positive impact on your energy field such as crystals, energy shields, and smudging. Create an altar with spiritual iconography that means something to you.

Spiritual Healers

Sometimes, spiritual imbalances such as those described above can only be addressed by a practitioner of exceptional spiritual knowledge, skill, and experience. A spiritual healer is often a person of faith, such as a rabbi, priest, monk, shaman or medicine man, yogi, or Tibetan lama. He might also be a person who possesses highly developed, psychic powers, such as a *feng shui* or *vastu shastra* practitioner, voodoo priest, dowser, psychic, intuitive, medium, or other spiritual master.

There are psychotherapists who specialize in resolving past life and spiritual possession issues through the use of regression therapy and hypnosis. There is also a specific acupuncture treatment for spiritual possession, although not every acupuncturist performs it.

Authentic spiritual healers are usually born with special gifts, exhibiting a heightened awareness, pure intentions, and the desire to develop their abilities over time with years of training and practice. Although everyone has clairvoyant ability,

6 MYTHS ABOUT ALTERNATIVE MEDICINE

more than potential is required to address complex spiritual issues in health.

You can develop insight by following the guidelines provided in Myth 1 for the development of an inner life, which will help alert you to a spiritual imbalance before it becomes a more serious problem. Detecting a spiritual problem, however, is different from resolving a spiritual problem. There are many types and levels of psychic ability as well as psychic resolution. It is not only important to find an authentic spiritual healer but also the right one for your needs.

Authentic spiritual healers capable of resolving complex spiritual issues are extremely difficult to find because their numbers are so few. They are certainly not found on television advertisements, infomercials, or by calling 900 telephone numbers. The spiritual healing profession is rife with charlatans and frauds, and some of them are very clever people.

There are spiritual healers who are well intentioned, but more often than not, their claims denote more wishful thinking and marketing skill than true psychic ability. Others may have psychic ability but are limited in what they can actually do for you. The heavy burden upon those who choose to participate in these practices as a path to healing is having to discern these differences in members of a profession who are notorious for telling people only what they want to hear.

Myth Six: Spirit is Always Positive

Although there may be few authentic spiritual healers who are qualified to address serious impediments to health, spiritual healing is a common and widely accepted practice in many diverse cultures around the world.

Keep an Open Mind

At first glance, a spiritual basis for health may seem absurd or inconsequential to the person who regards his spirituality as an object of suspicion or ridicule. Some things are true, however, whether you believe them or not. The fact is that people can and often do change their minds about spirituality after experiencing some sort of crisis in their lives.

In the event of a serious threat to your health, skepticism can quickly turn to optimism regarding consideration for all aspects of health and alternative paths to healing. Some people might characterize this newfound optimism as a desperation for answers, but it can also reflect openness, rediscovery, and ultimately growth.

Spiritual healing has become a lost art, in part, because it is not valued by science and technology-based medical systems. Unduly influenced by the latter, we have learned to be dismissive of experiences other than our own, especially ones we do not understand. However, almost everything that we now accept as a normal part of life began as someone else's farfetched notion—from the protestant church to the airplane.

Not so long ago, the bodymind connection, health benefits of nutritional supplements, and effect of diet on disease were all declared ridiculous by the same medical establishment that now embraces these same concepts today. One day, our spiritual connection to health will no doubt be rediscovered and accepted in the same manner and with the same ardor.

In one regard, spiritual healing has never left us, although we rarely hear about it. The Catholic church still quietly performs exorcisms. Due to the renewed interest in spiritual healing, the Church recently designated a Chicago priest to evaluate parishioners for this service. The book and movie *The Exorcist* was also based on a true story, which was published in *The Washington Post* in 1949, although the young boy's identity was never revealed.

Millions of dollars are spent on the study of the paranormal as well as the search for extraterrestrial life by reputable groups such as Harvard University's SETI Program (Search for Extraterrestrial Intelligence). Research studies have been conducted on the Near Death Experience (NDE), psychokinesis (the mind's ability to move objects), and the effect of spirituality and prayer on health. A new field of science termed neurotheology has also recently emerged, which investigates the brain patterns of altered states of consciousness.

Myth Six: Spirit is Always Positive

Spiritual healing is an important consideration in a holistic approach to alternative medicine. A belief in a spiritual basis for illness requires an open mind and a willingness to delve into unfamiliar territory. Exercise extreme caution before taking on a spiritual healing practice, and remember that the desire to explore spiritual aspects of your health does not absolve you from addressing physical and emotional impediments to health as well.

Guidelines for Resisting & Resolving a Spiritual Imbalance

1. Develop *personal health care power* (see Myth 1), and strengthen your spiritual immunity as described in this chapter.

2. Live your spirituality instead of talking about it.

3. Be open to new ideas and concepts about healing, including a spiritual basis for health.

4. Conduct extensive research into your options for spiritual healing.

5. Talk to people whom you trust about spiritual practices.

6. Choose spiritual healers carefully, and exercise caution when using their services. (See Myth 2.)

6 Myths About Alternative Medicine

Spirituality continues to grow as a primary social concern because of a renewed interest in the unexplainable and the search for greater meaning in our lives. Many of us have discovered that the pursuit of fame or fortune is not the cure. In fact, it may be what ails us because superficial pursuits such as these create more distress in our lives than they relieve. Fame and fortune may have been the goals of the past, but the care and cultivation of the soul are the goals of the future.

When getting our physical and emotional house in order, it behooves us to get our spiritual house in order to further the process of healing. It is important to consider the possibility of spiritual imbalance when dealing with any issue of health. Spiritual issues are at the core of true healing and their resolution will facilitate the success of all other alternative treatment therapies.

CONCLUSION

Two roads diverged in a wood, and I
I took the one less traveled by,
And that has made all the difference.

ROBERT FROST

Alternative medicine has many benefits if used properly. Alternative systems, methods, and techniques have been around for thousands of years, yet we late-blooming Westerners are only just discovering them. Although they do not always conform to our way of thinking and may seem strange on the surface, alternative medicine speaks to universal concepts and ideas that apply to any culture. We can benefit from the ancient wisdom that is the foundation for alternative medicine if we

6 MYTHS ABOUT ALTERNATIVE MEDICINE

are willing to assume some risks and make adjustments along the way.

It is important to understand the effect of translating a medicine from one culture into another, whose approach to health is very different from our own. Healing simply comes from within, not from another person, medicine, or external intervention. Within that knowledge lies great power for the health consumer.

Alternative providers are people, not gods, with the same problems, insecurities, misplaced motives, and misguided intentions as the rest of us. Ideally, they should have a different attitude and intention from their conventional medicine counterparts if they understand the true nature of healing and purpose of medicine, but this is not always the case. We should be unwilling to give up power to any health provider to the extent that it prevents us from doing the greater work necessary for healing.

Although there are guidelines for the manufacture and sale of alternative remedies and herbs, there are many products in the alternative marketplace that do not live up to their claims. The same remedies can differ enormously as to what they consist of and how they are made. Alternative remedies are also costly so we should either rely on the advice of a qualified herbalist or spend sufficient time educating ourselves about them and their differences in order get the most from their use.

Conclusion

We have developed an unhealthy dependence on science to tell us what to do and when to do it. This dependence permeates every aspect of our society and has stood unchallenged for decades. Few people are willing to publicly admit that science, in its current form, is both a limited tool and woefully inadequate to fully assess the inherent qualities of alternative medicine and their effect on the human body. The fact is that when we are more able to rely on and trust our own inherent knowledge, the need for traditional scientific validation will assume a more appropriate, supportive role in health care.

Common sense dictates that if something is taken from one culture and put into another culture with different values and priorities, the something will change. It would also then follow that if a medicine is taken from one culture and put into another culture with different values on and priorities for health and healing, the medicine will change. If the medicine is changed for the worse, its integrity is threatened along with its ability to work properly.

Instead of creating a new environment for the use of alternative medicine that is more compatible with its principles and values, we are naturally inclined to use it the same way we use conventional medicine. Substituting one medicine for another does not change the way we use medicine or our approach to health. If we do this, we must accept the fact that the effectiveness of alternative medicine

6 Myths About Alternative Medicine

will be compromised and the benefits available to us will be limited.

Alternative medicine makes conventional medicine better by making it more responsive to the needs of those it serves. Conventional medicine does not make alternative medicine better by institutionalizing and commercializing it. We must use alternative medicine with a totally different attitude and approach from the ones we use for conventional medicine, and we must insist that alternative providers do the same.

There are people who will always believe that spiritual aspects of health are not germane to any serious discussion about health or are only willing to consider them within a framework of what is positive and loving. This is an understandable outcome of a skeptical, fear-based society. But true healing will never be possible until we embrace all aspects of health.

We must open our hearts and minds to embrace all worlds of consciousness and existence and understand that good and bad and light and dark exist in everything. This realization will never come from another person but can only arise out of the pursuit of an inner life.

The coexistence of spiritual light and dark and the potential for spiritual imbalance are not new to religion and were once embraced by all ancient wisdom traditions. In Christianity, there still exists a strand of thought about these phenomena termed

Conclusion

Manichaeanism, which began with a third-century prophet named Mani. Manichaeanism flowed in and out of Christianity over the centuries and has also been affiliated with Buddhist practice. Although this tradition has an ominous connotation today, those who practice it generally believe in the reality of darkness and evil as basic tenants of the world along with a side by side existence of light and good.

Spiritual impediments to health are not easily resolved because of our lack of skill and experience in addressing these issues and the exceptional difficulty in finding authentic spiritual healers.

The importance of keeping an open mind is vital for anyone who wishes to use alternative medicine with any degree of success. There are many concepts in alternative medicine, such as the holistic concept of treating body, mind, and spirit as one, which may be unfamiliar to us. We typically do not open our minds or become motivated toward change until we face a crisis such as illness over which we feel we have little control.

Illness forces us to learn to be more comfortable with uncertainty because there is much wisdom to be gained from it. Within the words "I don't know" lies important knowledge about healing, along with an expanded capacity for compassion and love. It is through the insecurity and uncertainty of illness and

6 Myths About Alternative Medicine

other life challenges that our awareness is expanded and answers to larger problems often come to light.

It is important to consider the myths that surround alternative medicine and their influence upon us. Doing so in a constructive manner promotes its acceptance and responsible, safe, and effective use.

Always seek substance over superficiality when using alternative medicine in everything from choosing a healer or remedy to addressing all aspects of your health. It is incredible medicine. If you learn to use it in the manner in which it was originally intended, the possibility of true healing is within your immediate grasp.

BIBLIOGRAPHY

Ader, R., and N. Cohen. "Behaviorally Conditioned Immunosuppression." *Psychosomatic Medicine* 37 (July-Aug 1975): 333–40.

American Association of Poison Control Centers. "2001 Toxic Exposure Surveillance System Report." *American Journal of Emergency Medicine* 20 no. 5 (2002): 391–452.

Armstrong, Gregory L., Laura A. Conn, and Robert W. Pinner. "Trends in Infectious Disease Mortality in the United States During the 20th Century." *Journal of American Medical Association* 281 (January 6, 1999): 61–66.

Bateson, Gregory. *Mind And Nature*. New York: Bantam, 1979.

Beinfield, Harriet, and Efrem Korngold. *Between Heaven And Earth, A Guide To Chinese Medicine*. New York: Ballantine Books, 1991.

Benson, Herbert. *Timeless Healing—The Power and Biology of Belief*. New York: Simon and Schuster, 1997.

6 MYTHS ABOUT ALTERNATIVE MEDICINE

Berlin, Irving. "Anything You Can Do I Can Do Better," song from musical *Annie Get Your Gun*. New York, 1946.

Brunner, John. *Shockwave Rider*. New York: Ballantine Books, 1990.

Burke, Kenneth (1897–1993). *Permanence and Change*. New York: New Republic, 1935.

California Department of Health Services. Food and Drug Branch. *1997–1998 Compendium of Asian Patent Medicines*, 1998.

Center for Food Safety and Applied Nutrition. *Information Paper on L-tryptophan and 5-hydroxy-L-tryptophan*. Washington, D.C.: U.S. Food and Drug Administration, February 2001.

Daryai Lal Kapur. *Call Of The Great Master*. Punjab, India: Radha Soami Satsang Beas, 1964.

Einstein, Albert. *Out of My Later Years*. New York: Philosophical Library, Inc., 1950.

Flexner, Stuart, and Doris Flexner. *Wise Words and Wives Tales*. New York: Avon Books, 1993.

Fontanarosa, Phil B., and George D. Lundberg. "Alternative Medicine Meets Science." *New England Journal of Medicine* 280 (November 11, 1998): 1618–19.

Healthnotes® Online. Herb and remedy fact sheets [database online]. Portland, Oregon: Healthnotes, Inc. Available from http://www.healthnotes.com; INTERNET.

Bibliography

Hemingway, Ernest. *By-Line, Ernest Hemingway: Selected Articles and Dispatches of Four Decades*. Edited by William White. Carmichael, CA: Touchstone Books, 1998.

Hippocrene Books. *Hippocrates*. Translated by W.H.S. Jones. Cambridge, MA: Harvard University Press, 1923.

Kane, R.A., et al. "Everyday Matters in the Lives of Nursing Home Residents: Wish for and Perception of Choice and Control." *Journal of American Geriatric Society* 45 (September 1997): 1086–93.

Kennedy, John F. *Inaugural Address*. Boston: John F. Kennedy Library, January 20, 1961.

Kipling, Rudyard (1865–1936). *Barrack-Room Ballads*. Garden City, New York: Doubleday, Doran & Company, Inc., 1931.

Kirsch, Irving, and Guy Sapirstein. "Listening to Prozac but Hearing Placebo: A Meta-Analysis of Antidepressant Medication." *Prevention and Treatment* Vol. 1 (June 26, 1998). Available from http://www.journals.apa.org/prevention; INTERNET.

Lemley, Brad, "Heresy," *Discover*, August 2000.

Lowell, James Russell (1819–1891). *The Complete Poetical Works of James Russell Lowell*. Boston: Houghton, Mifflin, 1896.

National Center for Chronic Disease Prevention and Health Promotion. *Chronic Disease Overview*. Washington, D.C.: Centers for Disease Control and Prevention, August 30, 2002.

6 MYTHS ABOUT ALTERNATIVE MEDICINE

National Center for Complementary and Alternative Medicine. U.S. Department of Health and Human Services. *2003 Congressional Justification.* Silver Springs, Maryland: National Institutes of Health, 2003. Available from http://www.nccam.nih.gov/about/congressional/2003.pdf; INTERNET.

National Center for Complementary and Alternative Medicine. U.S. Department of Health and Human Services. *Alternative Medicine: Expanding Medical Horizons.* Silver Springs, Maryland: National Institutes of Health, 1993.

Niebuhr, Reinhold (1892–1971). *The Essential Reinhold Niebuhr: Selected Essays and Addresses.* New Haven, CT: Yale University Press, 1987.

NPD Group, Inc. *The 1998 Consumer Research Study on Book Purchasing.* Tarrytown, New York: American Booksellers Association, 1999.

Office of the Inspector General. *Adverse Event Reporting for Dietary Supplements: An Inadequate Safety Valve.* Washington, D.C: U.S. Department of Health and Human Services, 2001.

RavenWing, Josie. *The Book of Miracles.* Bloomington, Indiana: 1st Books, 2002.

Sheldrake, Rupert. *Dogs That Know When Their Owners Are Coming Home: and Other Unexplained Powers of Animals.* New York, New York: Three Rivers Press, 1999. (Add)

Stapleton, Stephanie. "Medicine's Chasm: The Wide Gulf Between Conventional and Alternative Approaches," *American Medical News,* June 3, 2002.

Bibliography

Syrus, Publilius (42 B.C.). *Minor Latin Poets.* Edited by E.H. Warmington and Translated by J. Wright Duff. Boston: Harvard University Press, 1935.

Talbot, Margaret, "The Placebo Prescription," *New York Times Magazine*, January 9, 2000.

Tierra, Michael. *The Way of Herbs.* Santa Cruz, California: Unity Press, 1980.

Tierra, Michael. "Standardized Herbal Extracts: An Herbalist's Perspective." *Natural Foods Merchandiser*, February 1999.

Tierra, Lesley. *The Herbs of Life.* Freedom, California: Crossing Press, 1992.

Wild, Russell, "Yoga, Inc.," *Yoga Journal*, November 2002.

Williamson, A.M., and Anne-Marie Feyer. "Moderate Sleep Deprivation Produces Impairments in Cognitive and Motor Performance Equivalent to Legally Prescribed Levels of Alcohol Intoxication." *Occupational and Environmental Medicine* 57 (October 2000): 649–55.

Woodward, Kenneth, Anne Underwood, and Donna Foote, "Is God Listening?" *Newsweek*, March 31, 1997.

Zava, David T. *Range of Progesterone Content of Body Creams.* San Leandro, California: Aeron LifeCycles, 1995.

INDEX

NOTE: Page numbers in *italics* indicate illustrations.

accessories and products,
        alternative, 57–58
acquisitionism, 134–35
addictions, 21, 126–28
alternative medicine/
        remedies. *See*
        remedies, alternative
alternative practices, 8, 66,
        117
alternative providers. *See also*
        healers/doctors
    and claims about curing,
        52–53
    and conventional
        medicine, 59–60, 168
    and dependency of
        patients/consumers, 9,
        49–52, 166
    dichotomy between
        Eastern points of view,
        and Western, 136–37
    and fees, 58–59
    and firsthand experiences,
        51, 67
    and gurus, 28–29, 67–68

and herbalists, 86–88, 166
and illnesses, 51–52
legitimacy of, 8, 48–49,
        52–62, 109
and physical, mental and
        spiritual trichotomy, 57
and point of view of
        conventional medicine,
        119–20, 123–29, 136–37,
        167–68
and professional training,
        60–61
and profits, 48–49, 50, 88
and single remedy/cure
        approach, 55–57
and source/facilitator of
        healing, 53–54
and spiritual healers,
        159–60, 163, 169
and spirituality, 62–63
and superficial approach
        to health care, 57–58,
        170
and symptoms, 56, 57
and time allowances for

healing process, 118–19
and timeliness of
improvement in health
condition, 62
and Western culture,
136–37
animal intuitiveness, 34
applied kinesiology/muscle
testing, 41
arginine remedy, 81
asthma, 131

Badell, Colleen *Is Your Health
Care Killing You?*, 31
beliefs
about healing process,
114–18, 137
about natural/gentle
nature of remedies,
9–10, 47, 48
and Eastern medical
practices, 116–18, 137
and prayer, 43, 106
vs. proof, 143
and Western culture, 99,
101, 114–16, 117
Berlin, Irving, 19
bodymind connection, 17,
21–23, 65, 162. *See also*
physical, mental and
spiritual trichotomy
Botanical Safety Handbook
(Herbal Products
Association), 85–86
Brunner, John, 94–95
Buddhism, 169. *See also*
Eastern medical
practices
Burke, Kenneth, 91

California Organic Foods Act
of 1990, 82

cartoon illustrations
aphrodisiac, herbal, *46*
fish cure, *24*
"perfect health," *90*
psychic, 142
ugly root remedy, *70*
yoga practices, *112*
Catholic Church, 14, 16, 147,
162, 168–69
Chinese patent medicines, 84
chronic illnesses, 21–22,
51–52
commercialization issues, 16,
18, 121–22, 143
competition, 18–19, 21, 133–34
conferences and workshops,
64–68
consciousness movement of
1960s, 21
control issues
and alternative practices,
117
and alternative remedies,
135
and conventional
medicine, 115
and dependency of
patients/consumers, 9,
42, 49–52, 166, 167
and egos, 35
and environmental issues,
15, 17, 101–3, 129
and government
regulations, 82–83
and healing process, 11, 151
and illnesses, 25, 169
and inner life,
development of, 37
and negative thoughts/
actions, 158
and patriarchal point of
view, 13

178

Index

and responsibility for
personal health, 30,
32, 44, 60, 68–69, 122,
131–32
and scientific studies, 92,
97, 100
and self-diagnosis, 115
and Western culture, 37,
55, 101, 102
conventional medicine. *See
also* healers/doctors
and alternative providers,
59–60, 168
alternative remedies
compared with, 8–9,
21–22
and control issues, 115
and excessive use of
medicine, 115–16
and fast-acting invasive
therapies, 21
and healing process, 21, 42
and health care process,
20–21, 57–58, 119–20,
123–29
history of, 13–17
hormone replacement
therapy (HRT), 97
and identity issues, 20
and immune system, 104
and integration with
alternative remedies,
110–11
and placebo effect, 105
point of view of, 119–20,
123–29, 136–37, 167–68
and profits, 98
and providers,
conventional, 9, 42,
49–52, *90*, 167
and scientific studies, 10,
14, 94–98, 167

and silicone breast
implants, 116
steroid remedy, 116
cost issues, and fees of
alternative providers,
58–59. *See also*
profitability issues

dependency issues, 9, 42,
49–52, 166, 167
depression, 130
DHEA remedy, 85
diagnosis issues
and diagnosable
conditions, 116
and self-diagnosis, 63–64,
115
Dietary Supplement Health
and Education Act of
1994 (DSHEA), 82
diseases. *See* illnesses
dowsing techniques, 41

Eastern medical practices.
See also remedies,
alternative
and allowing proper time
for, 118–19
and application to
Western culture, 10,
113–14
and beliefs about healing
process, 116–18, 137
and consciousness
movement of 1960s, 21
and dichotomy with
Western point of view,
136–37
and imbalance, spiritual,
117–18
and interdependence with
healers/medicine, 117

6 Myths About Alternative Medicine

and layers of healing,
117–19
and maintenance of
health, 117
and surrender to
experiences, 44
echinacea remedy, 74
economic issues, and fees of
alternative providers,
58–59. *See also*
profitability issues
education issues, 60–61,
63–68, 89, 166
Einstein, Albert, 108–9
End of Science, The (Horgan),
10
environmental issues, 15, 17,
101–3, 129
ephedra remedy, 64
Exorcist, The (film), 162

faith
in higher power, 106, 151
and physical, mental and
spiritual trichotomy,
107, 110
and placebo effect, 105
power of, 104–7
prayer and beliefs, 43, 106
scientific studies, and
synthesis with, 101–3
spirituality of, 98–99
and trust in personal
judgment, 32, 69, 93,
106–8, 109
fate, 146, 151
female issues, 96, 97, 116
Food, Drug and Cosmetic
Act, 82
Food and Drug
Administration (FDA),
64, 82
Frost, Robert, 165

ginko remedy, 85
government regulations
and control issues, 82–83
U.S. Department of
Agriculture, 82
U.S. Food and Drug
Administration (FDA),
64, 82
U.S. Poison Control
Centers, 64
gurus, 28–29, 67–68

healers/doctors. *See also*
alternative providers;
conventional medicine:
and providers,
conventional; inner
life, development of
Healer always knows best
(Myth 1), 25–45
and active role by
patients/consumers,
29–31, 42, 44–45
and beliefs, 43
and dependency of
patients/consumers, 9,
42, 49–52, 166, 167
and egos, 35
gurus, 28–29
and healing practices,
spiritual, 34–36, 106,
157–59, 160, 163
and healing process, 26,
42
and inner life,
development of, 33–34
intentions of, 131–36
and interdependence of
patients/consumers,
25–28, 42, 139
and limitations for
change by patients/
consumers, 54–55

180

Index

and muscle testing/
applied kinesiology, 41
and passive/submissive
approach of patients,
25–26, 27, 32, 42
and personal health care
power, 29–31, 42, 45,
109, 163
and prayer, 43
and responsibility for
personal health care,
30, 32, 44, 60, 68–69,
122, 131–32
and surrender to
experiences, 43–45
and Wizard of Oz , 25
healing practices, spiritual,
34–36, 106, 157–59, 160,
163
healing process
and active role by
patients/consumers in,
29–31, 42, 44–45
and ambiguity, 99, 101,
116, 117
and animal intuitiveness,
34
and beliefs, 114–18, 137
and control issues, 11, 151
and conventional
medicine, 21, 42
and detachment of
patients/consumers,
115–16
Eastern medical practices,
and beliefs about,
116–18, 137
and healers/doctors, 26,
42
holistic approach to,
21–23, 51–52, 124–25,
144, 168–69
and illnesses, 117–18

and individual differences
of patients/consumers,
26, 95–96, 99–100, 118
and inner life,
development of, 33–34
and interdependence of
patients/consumers,
25–28, 42, 117, 139
and layers of healing,
117–19
and personal health care
power, 29–31, 42, 45,
109, 163
positive and negative in,
143–44, 146–47, 151–52,
154, 168–69
and self-help industry, 26
and spirit/spirituality,
144, 145–46, 152–54,
160–64, 168–69
and symptoms, 20
and time allowances for,
118–19
and timeliness of
improvement in health
condition, 62
and trust in personal
judgment, 32, 69, 93,
106–8, 109
vs. fast-acting invasive
therapies, 21
Western culture, and
beliefs about, 99, 101,
114–16, 117
health care process
and conventional
medicine, 20–21, 57–58,
119–20, 123–29
superficial approach to,
57–58, 119–20, 131–36,
170
health issues. *See* illnesses
herbalists, 86–88, 166

Herbal Products Association, *Botanical Safety Handbook,* 85–86
herbal remedies, *46,* 71, 74–77, 83, 85–86, 88
higher power, 106, 151
Hindu beliefs. *See* Eastern medical practices
Hippocrates, 29, 118
holistic approach to healing process, 21–23, 51–52, 124–25, 144, 168–69
Horgan, John *The End of Science,* 10
hormone replacement therapy (HRT), 97
hormones, female, 96, 97

identity issues
and conventional medicine, 20
and healers/doctors, 28–29, 67–68
illnesses
and alternative providers, 51–52
and alternative remedies, 82–83, 86, 138–39
and ambiguity in healing process, 99, 101, 116, 117
asthma, 131
and bodymind connection, 17, 21–23, 65, 162
cartoon about, *90*
causes of, 117–18, 150–52
chronic illnesses, 21–22, 51–52
and control issues, 25, 169
depression, 130
and diagnosable conditions, 116

and female hormonal fluctuations, 96
and healing process, 117–18
and holistic approach to healing process, 21–23, 51–52, 124–25, 144, 168–69
and imbalance, spiritual, 117–18, 156, 157, 164, 169
and immune system, 104
and lifestyles, 130–31
life-threatening, 51–52
and maintaining health, 12
and nature of health, 11–12
as opportunities for learning and growth, 12
parasites, 130–31
and responsibility for personal health, 30, 32, 44, 60, 68–69, 122, 131–32
and scientific studies, 102–3
sleep disorders, 96
and spirit/spirituality, 150–52, 169–70
and timeliness of improvement in health condition, 62
imbalance, spiritual, 117–18, 156, 157, 164, 169
immune system, 104
immunity, spiritual, 156, 158–59
inner life. *See also* spirit/ spirituality
and control issues, 37
development of, 37–40

Index

and dowsing techniques,
41
and healing process,
33–34
and intuition, 34–37
and love, 37
and muscle testing/
applied kinesiology, 41
and silence, 36–37, 39,
149, 153
and surrender to
experiences, 43–45
intentions of healers/
doctors, 131–36
interdependence issues,
25–28, 42, 117, 139
intimacy issues, 18–21
intuition, 34–37, 106
*Is Your Health Care Killing
You?* (Badell), 31

*Journal of the American
Medical Association*
(JAMA), 92

kava kava remedy, 84
kinesiology, applied, 41
Kipling, Rudyard, 113

lifestyle issues, 129–31
love, and development of
inner life, 37
Lowell, James Russell, 113
L-tryptophan remedy, 84

Manichaeanism, 169
materialism issues, 132,
134–35, 136, 148–50
mindbody connection, 17,
21–23, 65, 162. *See also*
physical, mental and
spiritual trichotomy
Muir, John, 23

muscle testing/applied
kinesiology, 41
Muslim beliefs. *See* Eastern
medical practices
myths
All remedies are created
equal (Myth 3), 71–89
Healer always knows best
(Myth 1), 25–45
It can't hurt you (Myth 2),
47–69
It's a good substitute for
conventional medicine
(Myth 5), 113–41
Spirit is always positive
(Myth 6), 143–64
You can't use it without
proof (Myth 4), 91–111

National Institutes of Health,
91
negative aspects
and healing process,
143–44, 146–47, 151–52,
154, 168–69
and negative thoughts/
actions, 158
"New Age" phenomenon,
48, 64–68, 126–28
Niebuhr, Reinhold, 43

paranormal/supernatural
events, 155, 162
parasites, 130–31
patients/consumers
and active role in healing
process, 29–31, 42,
44–45
and cartoons about, *90,
112*
and dependency on
health providers, 9,
49–52, 166

6 Myths About Alternative Medicine

and detachment from
  healing process, 115–16
and education about
  alternative remedies,
  63–64, 89, 166
and effective use of
  alternative remedies,
  139–42, 165, 166
and gurus, 28–29
and individual
  differences, 26, 95–96,
  99–100, 118
and interdependence with
  alternative providers,
  25–28, 42, 117, 139
and lifestyles, 129–31
and limitations for
  change, 54–55
and New Age
  phenomenon, 48,
  64–68, 126–28
objectification of, 114–15
and open minded
  approach to spirit/
  spirituality, 156,
  161–63, 169
passive/submissive
  approach of, 25–26, 27,
  32, 42
and personal health care
  power, 29–31, 42, 45,
  109, 163
profits, and rights of, 50
and responsibility for
  personal health care,
  30, 32, 44, 60, 68–69,
  122, 131–32
rights of, 33, 50
and scientific studies,
  choices about, 100–101
and self-diagnosis, 63–64,
  115

and trust in personal
  judgment, 32, 69, 93,
  106–8, 109
patriarchal point of view, 13
physical, mental and
  spiritual trichotomy.
  See also spirit/
  spirituality
  and alternative providers,
  57
  and alternative remedies,
  89, 99
  and bodymind
  connection, 17, 21–23,
  65, 162
  and faith, 107, 110
  and holistic approach to
  healing process, 21–23,
  51–52, 124–25, 144,
  168–69
  and illnesses, causes of,
  117–18, 150–52
  and patriarchal point of
  view, 13
  and spirit/spirituality,
  146, 154–55
  and spirituality, 62–63
  and Western culture, 12,
  13–14, 16–19, 121–22,
  143
placebo effect, 105
positive aspects
  in healing process,
  143–44, 146–47, 151–52,
  154, 168–69
  Spirit is always positive
  (Myth 6), 143–64
  and spirit/spirituality,
  143, 144, 146
power
  of faith, 104–7
  higher power, 106, 151

Index

personal health care
power, 29–31, 42, 45,
109, 163
of suggestion, 105
and Wizard of Oz, 25
practices. *See also* Eastern
medical practices
alternative practices, 8,
66, 117
psychology practices, 16
spiritual healing practices,
34–37, 106, 157–59, 160,
163
spiritual practices, 145,
149, 150, 169
yoga practices, *112,* 128,
133
prayer and beliefs, 43, 106
professional training, 60–61.
See also education
issues
profitability issues
and alternative providers,
48–49, 50, 88
and alternative remedies,
7, 8, 48, 50, 121–23
and conventional
medicine, 98
and conventional
providers, 50
and New Age events, 66
and patients/consumers
rights, 50
and self-help industry,
26
progesterone remedy, 84
providers. *See* alternative
providers;
conventional medicine:
and providers,
conventional
psychology practices, 16

religious issues. *See also* faith;
inner life, development
of; physical, mental
and spiritual
trichotomy
and Catholic Church, 14,
16, 162, 168–69
and spirit/spirituality,
147, 148
remedies, alternative. *See
also* Eastern medical
practices; faith; spirit/
spirituality
It can't hurt you (Myth 2),
47–69
All remedies are created
equal (Myth 3), 71–89
You can't use it without
proof (Myth 4), 91–111
It's a good substitute for
conventional medicine
(Myth 5), 113–41
and acquisitionism, 134–35
administration of, 71
arginine remedy, 81
and baths, 77, 81
and beauty treatments, 77
and capsules, 77–78
cartoons about, *24, 46, 70,*
142
and Chinese patent
medicines, 84
and chronic use, 85
and claims about cures,
85–86, 89, 166
commercialization of,
121–22
compared with
conventional medicine,
8–9, 21–22
and competition issues,
133–34

185

complexity of, 72–73
and control issues, 135
conventional point of
   view, and use of,
   119–20, 123–29, 136–37,
   167–68
and conventional
   providers, 50
cost of, 88, 166
and dangerous
   ingredients, 83, 84–86
DHEA remedy, 85
and dietary supplements,
   82–83
and dosages, 86, 89
echinacea remedy, 74
effectiveness of, 7, 11–12,
   47–49, 71, 89, 108
effective use of, 139–42,
   165, 166
and elitism, 58, 123
and emotions, 108, 109
ephedra remedy, 64
ginko remedy, 85
and government
   regulations, 82–83
guidelines for choosing
   and using, 88–89
and herbalists, 86–88, 166
and herbs, 46, 71, 74–77,
   83, 85–86, 88
and holistic approach to
   healing process, 21–23,
   51–52, 124–25, 144,
   168–69
and illnesses, 82–83, 86,
   138–39
and individual
   differences, 26, 95–96,
   99–100, 118
and ingredients, 85
institutionalization of,
   120–23

and integration with
   conventional medicine,
   110–11
and intentions of healers/
   doctors, 131–36
and interactions, adverse,
   83, 84, 86, 89
and intuition, 34–37, 106
and juices, 79
kava kava remedy, 84
and legitimacy of
   alternative practices, 8
and lifestyles, 129–31
and liquid tinctures, 76, 78
locations for purchasing,
   72–73
L-tryptophan remedy, 84
and manufacturing
   information, 83, 166
and manufacturing
   processes, 71, 76–77,
   166
and materialism, 132,
   134–35, 136
and medical allergies, 86
misconceptions about, 11
natural/gentle medicine
   beliefs about, 9–10,
   47, 48
and New Age
   phenomenon, 48,
   64–68, 126–28
and oils, 77, 80
and over-the-counter
   distribution, 83
and patients/consumers
   education, 63–64, 89,
   166
and physical, mental and
   spiritual trichotomy,
   89, 99
and placebo effect, 105
and powders, 77, 79

186

Index

and power of suggestion,
105
and pregnancy, 86
and profits, 7, 8, 48, 50,
121–23
progesterone remedy, 84
and proof, 143
and psyche, 98
and reactions, adverse, 85
and regulations, 48
and responsibility for
health, 30, 32, 44, 60,
68–69, 122, 131–32
and sacredness of all
things, 13
and salves, 79
and scientific studies, 10,
91–94, 95, 107–8, 109
selection of, 71–72, 81–82
and self-diagnosis, 63–64
single remedy/cure
approach, 55–57
social acceptability of, 7,
8, 22
and social issues, 135–36
and soups, 80
St. John's wort remedy,
10, 84, 130
and standardized
formulas, 75–76
and superficial approach
to health care, 57–58,
119–20, 131–36, 170
and suppositories, 80–81
and symptoms, 8, 21, 62
and syrups, 80
and tablets/pills, 78
and teas, 79
and time allowances for
healing process, 118–19
and timeliness of
improvement in health
condition, 62

types of, 72
valerian remedy, 85
and Western culture,
application to, 10,
113–14, 167

scientific studies
and alternative remedies,
10, 91–94, 95, 107–8,
109
and control issues, 92, 97,
100
and conventional
medicine, 10, 14, 94–98,
167
faith, and synthesis with,
101–3
and illnesses, 102–3
patients/consumers, and
choices about, 100–101
self-diagnosis, 63–64, 115
self-help industry, 26
Serenity Prayer, 43
silence, and development of
inner life, 36–37, 39,
149, 153
silicone breast implants, 116
sleep disorders, 96
social issues. *See* Western
culture
spirit/spirituality. *See*
also faith; inner life,
development of;
physical, mental and
spiritual trichotomy
Spirit is always positive
(Myth 6), 143–64
and alternative providers,
62–63
and applied spirituality, 150
commercialization of, 143
and connectdness,
spiritual, 152

187

definition of, 146–48
and ego, role of, 151, 152
of faith, 98–99
and fate, 146, 151
and healers, spiritual, 159–60, 163, 169
and healing, spiritual, 152–54, 160–64
and healing practices, 34–37, 106, 157–59, 160, 163
and healing process, 144, 145–46, 152–54, 160–64, 168–69
and illnesses, 150–52, 169–70
and imbalance, spiritual, 117–18, 156, 157, 164, 169
and immunity, spiritual, 156, 158–59
and materialism, spiritual, 148–50
negative in, 143–44, 146–47, 151–52, 154, 168–69
open minded approach to, 156, 161–63, 169
and physical, mental and spiritual trichotomy, 146, 154–55
and physical world, 154
positive in, 143, 144, 146
and religious issues, 147, 148
and spirituality issues, 62–63, 150
and spiritual practices, 145, 149, 150, 169
and spirit world issues, 154–56
superficial approach to, 148, 150

vs. regret, feelings of, 151
in Western culture, 10–11, 92–93, 144–46
spiritual practices, 145, 149, 150, 169
St. John's wort remedy, 10, 84, 130
steroid remedy, 116
superficiality issues
    in alternative practices, 66
    and alternative remedies, use of, 131–36
    and spirit/spirituality, 148, 150
    in use of alternative remedies, 57–58, 119–20, 170
    and Western culture, 101, 164
supernatural/paranormal events, 155, 162
surrender to experiences, 43–45
symptoms
    and alternative providers, 56, 57
    and alternative remedies, 8, 21, 62
    and healing process, 20
    and Western culture, 8, 57, 115, 116
Syrus, Publilius, 71

technology, modern, 20, 103
time issues
    and time allowances for healing process, 118–19
    and timeliness of improvement in health condition, 62

U.S. Department of Agriculture, 82

Index

U.S. Food and Drug
Administration (FDA),
64, 82
U.S. Poison Control Centers,
64

valerian remedy, 85

Washington Post, The, 162
Western culture. *See also*
conventional medicine
and alternative providers,
136–37
alternative remedies,
and application to, 10,
113–14, 167
beliefs about healing
process, 99, 101,
114–16, 117
and commercialization
issues, 16, 18, 121–22,
143
and control issues, 37, 55,
101, 102
and diagnosable
conditions, 116
and dichotomy of Eastern
point of view, 136–37
Eastern medical practices,
and application to, 10,
113–14

and intentions of healers/
doctors, 131–36
and intimacy issues,
18–21
and patriarchal point of
view, 13
and physical, mental and
spiritual trichotomy,
12, 13–14, 16–19,
121–22, 143
and regret, feelings of, 151
and spirit/spirituality,
10–11, 92–93, 144–46
superficiality of, 101, 164
and surrender to
experiences, 44
and symptoms, 8, 57, 115,
116
technology, modern, 103
and technology, modern,
20
and yoga practices, 128
Western medicine. *See*
conventional medicine
Wizard of Oz, 25
women's issues, 96, 97, 116
workshops and conferences,
64–68

yoga practices, *112,* 128, 133